PUBLIC HEALTH IN THE 21ST CENTURY

PHYSICAL THERAPY: THEORY, PRACTICES AND BENEFITS

PUBLIC HEALTH IN THE 21ST CENTURY

Additional books in this series can be found on Nova's website under the Series tab.

Additional E-books in this series can be found on Nova's website under the E-books tab.

REHABILITATIVE TECHNOLOGY, TREATMENT AND PRACTICE

Additional books in this series can be found on Nova's website under the Series tab.

Additional E-books in this series can be found on Nova's website under the E-books tab.

PUBLIC HEALTH IN THE 21ST CENTURY

PHYSICAL THERAPY: THEORY, PRACTICES AND BENEFITS

JAMES P. BENNETT
EDITOR

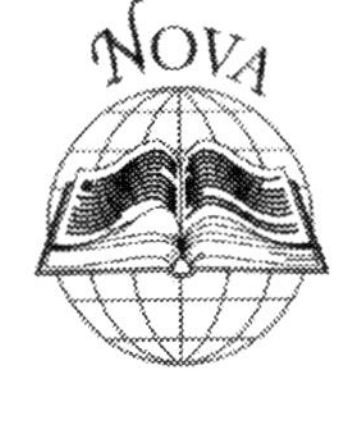

Nova Science Publishers, Inc.
New York

For permission to use material from this book please contact us:
Telephone 631-231-7269; Fax 631-231-8175
Web Site: http://www.novapublishers.com

LIBRARY OF CONGRESS CATALOGING-IN-PUBLICATION DATA

Physical therapy : theory, practices, and benefits / editor, James P. Bennett.
p. ; cm.
Includes bibliographical references and index.
ISBN 978-1-61122-418-4 (hardcover)
1. Physical therapy. I. Bennett, James P., 1960-
[DNLM: 1. Physical Therapy Modalities. 2. Pain--therapy. WB 460]
RM700.P475 2010
615.8'2--dc22
2010041310

Published by Nova Science Publishers, Inc. † New York

CONTENTS

PREFACE

Physical therapy is a health profession that assesses and provides treatment to individuals to develop, maintain and restore maximum movement and function throughout life. This includes providing treatment in circumstances where movement and function are threatened by aging, injury, disease or environmental factors. This important book presents current research in the study of physical therapy including: therapies and motor function assessments in chronic pain syndromes; fibromyalgia syndrome; breathing pattern disorders in physical therapy; home-based shoulder rehabilitation; isokinetic strengthening in multiple sclerosis patients; and traditional mirror therapy (TMT) in the physical therapy management of movement and postural control problems.

Chapter 1 - Introduction. Longstanding pain syndromes are among the greatest threats to health and welfare in the western world. The etiologies of these syndromes are often complex and unclear. For instance, chronic pelvic pain (CPP) is affecting up to 4% of all women, leading to excess therapies, and even futile surgical interventions. In the context of contemporary approaches to assessments of motor functions and therapeutic interventions, the authors present the results of a novel approach to assessment (Standardized Mensendieck Test, SMT) and a hybrid of Mensendieck physical therapy and cognitive psycho-therapy: somatocogntitive therapy.

Methods. 40 women with CPP (average age 32.3 years) were recruited from the Department of Obstetrics and Gynecology of a tertiary care teaching hospital, and randomized into two groups (control and intervention). The intervention consisted of somatocognitive therapy, 1 session per week for 12 weeks. At inclusion (baseline), after 3 months and after 1 year the women were assessed for motor patterns (using SMT), pain load (using a visual analogue scale of pain, VAS) and for psychological distress (using the general health questionnaire, GHQ 30).

Results. The intervention group showed significant ($p < 0.01$) improvement for motor patterns (up to 71% increase in SMT scores), pain load (up to 64% reduction in VAS scores) and psychological distress (up to 36% reduction in GHQ-30 scores), as well as increased coping, compared to the control group. 9 months after end of therapy, the outcomes were improved as compared to end of therapy scores.

Conclusions. The results demonstrate that somatocognitive therapy is efficient in improving motor function, pain load and psychological distress in women with CPP. The further reduction in symptom load after therapy may indicate that the women had been given tools through therapy that they could utilize in daily living outside of therapy. The outcomes of this study are discussed in light of contemporary approaches to therapy in longstanding pain syndromes.

Chapter 2 - Patients with fibromyalgia syndrome (FS) experience variable persistent pain, yet causes of episodic pain flares are often inexplicable. Stress has been suggested as a trigger, however reported correlations between pain intensity and same-day stress are low. Several recent FS case studies report notable increases in pain ten days following stressful episodes. This study's purpose was to assess the impact of stress across time on latent pain intensity changes as well as sensory and affective pain responses in a larger FS patient sample. Thirty-eight patients with FS admitted to a four-week multi-disciplinary pain program completed the following inventories daily for 4 weeks: Daily Stress Inventory (DSI), Visual Analog Scale (VAS) for pain intensity, McGill Pain Questionnaire Short Form (MPQSF). Affective (MPQSF-A) and sensory (MPQSF-S) pain scores from the MPQSF were analyzed separately. Serial-lag correlations between DSI and VAS, MPQSF-S, and MPQSF-A assessed the impact of daily stress across time on the intensity, sensory, and affective response to episodic pain flares. Since 35 of 38 participants rated the intake/initial evaluation day of the program as the most stressful day of their four week stay in the program, three separate one-way repeated measures ANOVAs were conducted to compare VAS, MGQSF-A, MGQSF-S scores for each day of participation (up to 14 days) following the stressful initial intake day. Pain intensity, sensory, and affective scores yielded very low correlations with same-day stress. However, serial-lag correlations revealed significant relationships between high stress days and pain flares occurring ten days later for pain intensity ($r=+0.53$), pain sensation ($r=+0.46$), and affective responses ($r=+0.59$). Based on ANOVA with Bonferroni correction, VAS scores yielded significant points at 3, 10, and 13 days following program intake. MGSFQ-S yielded a significant point 10 days following intake. MGSFQ-A yielded significant points at 10 and 13 days following intake. In all statistical comparisons, the most significant mean elevations in pain responses occurred on day 10 following program intake/ initial evaluation. It may be concluded that stress increases are associated with delayed episodic pain flares and pronounced sensory and affective responses to pain occurring ten days later in patients with FS.

Chapter 3 - While body norms such as body temperature, heart rate and blood pressure, and lung volumes are routinely measured by health practitioners, breathing patterns are usually overlooked. Breathing pattern refers not only to lung function and respiration, but also to biomechanics and motor control. In particular, clinical observations of rate and depth of breaths per minute, and patterns of breathing - i.e. nose versus mouth and upper chest versus the energy efficient diaphragm. However, it is important to note that there is so much more to breathing in and out than a nose/diaphragm pattern in the treatment and assessment of breathing pattern disorders. Breathing is one of our most vital functions and a disordered breathing pattern can be the first sign that all is not well, whether it be biomechanically, physiologically or psychologically. For example: breathing rapidly sharply reduces blood carbon dioxide levels. The shift in carbon dioxide chemistry (hypocapnia) may cause physiological changes in the body leading to muscle fatigue, spasm (tetany) and pain.

Breathing pattern disorders affect people of all ages and stages in the population, and appear in all areas of clinical practice. They cause widespread distress and anxiety to the individual, their families and friends, as well as causing high costs to communities in days lost from school or work, and to the healthcare system itself. Physiotherapeutic strategies have been used since the early 1960's in the treatment of breathing pattern disorders in both people with organic lung disease and those without. Cardiorespiratory physiotherapy is well established within the orthodox medical literature - assessment and treatment regimes contain components of breathing education and retraining.

The focus of this chapter will be on the emerging area of musculoskeletal physiotherapy and breathing pattern disorders. Physiotherapists are ideally placed to recognise and treat these disorders, both within the public health and private healthcare systems.

Chapter 4 - Formal post-operative physical therapy is the standard of care following shoulder surgeries to include arthroscopic reconstructions, decompressions, rotator cuff repairs, and arthroplasties. A significant amount of health care resources are spent on these rehabilitation programs, however their cost-effectiveness and necessity have not been established.

A retrospective analysis conducted of 2 consecutive groups of patients undergoing total shoulder arthroplasty (TSA) for primary osteoarthritis is reviewed. One group was treated with formal physical therapy (PT), and one group was treated with home-based, physician-guided PT. ASES and Simple Shoulder Test (SST) scores significantly improved in both groups at all follow-up periods. Forward flexion and abduction were significantly improved in the home-based group at all time points, whereas an initial improvement in forward flexion and abduction in the formal PT group was lost at final follow-up. There were no significant differences in final ASES or SST scores between groups at final follow-up. However, forward flexion, abduction, and the Short Form-36 physical component summary scores in the home-based group were significantly better than those patients with formal PT at final follow-up. No significant improvements in internal rotation or SF-36 mental component summary were seen within or between the groups at final follow-up. Overall, there was no difference in patient satisfaction.

A home-based, physician-guided therapy program may provide adequate rehabilitation after TSA, allowing for a reduction in cost for the total procedure. Based on these results, the authors have developed home therapy programs for shoulder surgeries to include arthroscopic procedures in addition to arthroplasties. By focusing on patient-oriented, home-based therapy programs, they allow patients to take full responsibility for their recovery and not rely on an outside agency to be responsible for their result. Based on the early results it is suggested that this approach works well for many patients, however, supervised PT may still be required for patients who are not progressing as expected. Close physician follow-up and referral to formal PT may be necessary for patients who are not able to meet rehabilitation guidelines on their own. Better collaboration between PT and surgeons can lead to better clinical outcomes, but further studies with valid evaluation of outcome data are necessary.

Chapter 5 - Muscle weakness is a main factor of neurological impairment in several disease such multiple sclerosis, cerebral palsy or stroke patients. Several studies have stressed the interest of muscle strength training in such a situation with functional improvement. Reliable and reproducible, isokinetic evaluation can quantify the motor deficit and guide the strength training of muscle groups. The weakness of hamstring muscle seems crucial in reducing the walking speed regardless of the level of deficit that of the quadriceps for a disability becomes greater. The isokinetic strengthening of the muscle groups with no consequence on spasticity provides significant functional results. In multiple sclerosis, regular muscular strengthening allows to maintain or even improve their functional level. In this situation, the isokinetic strengthening seems relevant. After an isokinetic evaluation allowing the assessment of the patient's deficits, a protocol of rehabilitation including strength training is defined. Three protocols are identified. The first one takes care of the recurvatum of the knee, the second allows an intensification of quadriceps and the third one is specific of hip flexors. This isokinetic training which is associated with a standard multidisciplinary approach shows an important functional interest including: transfer, climb and descent of staircases, improvements of gait (speed, quality and endurance). However, it seems important and necessary to have a regular follow up because of the evolution of the disease.

Chapter 6 - Mirrors have a long history as an 'essential' piece of rehabilitation equipment, and can be found in many physical therapy treatment areas. Traditionally one of their main uses is to provide patients with a reflected body image of themselves, usually as (a component of) a therapeutic strategy aimed at retraining movement control and posture. For example, when as a result of central nervous system (CNS) damage such as stroke, people have impaired postural control, then therapists might provide them within a reflected mirror image of themselves to deliver augmented visual feedback during treatment sessions where motor training is occurring.

There has recently been much interest in the therapeutic use of mirrors placed perpendicular to the patient's coronal plane; i.e mirrors able to reflect an image of one limb onto the limb of the opposite body side. Recent works by researchers such as Ramachandran [1-4], and Sutbeyaz and Yavuzer [5, 6], have indicated that this may be a useful therapeutic strategy in instances where CNS pathology has resulted in unilateral instances of paresis, neglect or phantom pain. So for example, a mirror might be used to reflect the left (sound) arm onto the right (paralysed) arm following a stroke, as part of a therapeutic strategy aiming to rehabilitate movement on the affected side. One proposed mechanism is that reflection creates an illusion of normal movement/sensation on the affected side of the body, thus facilitating voluntary production of movement and/or normal sensory processing on that side.

In: Physical Therapy
Editor: James P. Bennett

ISBN: 978-1-61122-418-4

Chapter 1

THERAPIES AND MOTOR FUNCTION ASSESSMENTS IN LONGSTANDING PAIN SYNDROMES: THE EFFECT OF SOMATOCOGNITIVE THERAPY IN A RANDOMIZED, CONTROLLED INTERVENTION STUDY OF WOMEN WITH CHRONIC PELVIC PAIN

***Gro Killi Haugstad*[*1] *and Tor S. Haugstad*[≠2]**

[1]Oslo University College, Department of Health Science, Pilestredet, Oslo, Norway

[2]Sunnaas National Rehabilitation Hospital, Departments of Neurorehabilitation and Research, Nesoddtangen, Norway

ABSTRACT

Introduction. Longstanding pain syndromes are among the greatest threats to health and welfare in the western world. The etiologies of these syndromes are often complex and unclear. For instance, chronic pelvic pain (CPP) is affecting up to 4% of all women, leading to excess

---

* e-mail: grokilli.haugstad@hf.hio.no, phone # +47 22 45 24 40

≠ e-mail: tor.haugstad@sunnaas.no, phone # +47 911 53 516

therapies, and even futile surgical interventions. In the context of contemporary approaches to assessments of motor functions and therapeutic interventions, we present the results of a novel approach to assessment (Standardized Mensendieck Test, SMT) and a hybrid of Mensendieck physical therapy and cognitive psychotherapy: somato-cogntitive therapy.

Methods. 40 women with CPP (average age 32.3 years) were recruited from the Department of Obstetrics and Gynecology of a tertiary care teaching hospital, and randomized into two groups (control and intervention). The intervention consisted of somatocognitive therapy, 1 session per week for 12 weeks. At inclusion (baseline), after 3 months and after 1 year the women were assessed for motor patterns (using SMT), pain load (using a visual analogue scale of pain, VAS) and for psychological distress (using the general health questionnaire, GHQ 30).

Results. The intervention group showed significant ($p < 0.01$) improvement for motor patterns (up to 71% increase in SMT scores), pain load (up to 64% reduction in VAS scores) and psychological distress (up to 36% reduction in GHQ-30 scores), as well as increased coping, compared to the control group. 9 months after end of therapy, the outcomes were improved as compared to end of therapy scores.

Conclusions. The results demonstrate that somatocognitive therapy is efficient in improving motor function, pain load and psychological distress in women with CPP. The further reduction in symptom load after therapy may indicate that the women had been given tools through therapy that they could utilize in daily living outside of therapy. The outcomes of this study are discussed in light of contemporary approaches to therapy in longstanding pain syndromes.

Chronic Pelvic Pain

Chronic pelvic pain (CPP) in women[1] is defined as lower abdominal pain unrelated to pregnancy that has lasted for at least six months. The pain may be described as dull aching, sharp, cramping or a feeling of painful pressure or heaviness deep within the pelvis. Pain during intercourse is rather common, and some also report experiencing pain while having a bowel movement, while lifting heavy burdens or even during the performance of simple movements of normal daily life activities, such as sitting down, and even while

[1] Medically unexplained chronic pain in the pelvic area also occurs in males (Cornel et al. 2005, FitzGerald 2005, Anderson et al. 2005, 2006, and Giubilei et al. 2007). "Prostatitis" is an alternative diagnosis sometimes used for CPP in males (Bergman & Zeitlin 2007). We have not addressed CPP in male patients in this study.

walking and standing. It may be relieved while lying down, and particularly so while taking a hot tub bath. The patients often think that the origin of the pain is a disease or dysfunction in the genital organs such as the uterus or the ovaries. The majority claim that the pain is the worst during the second part of the menstrual cycle. Pollakisuria may occur and some degree of menstrual disturbance is not uncommon. However, pain occurring *exclusively* around menstruation (dysmenorrhoea) or with intercourse (dyspareunia) is excluded from the definition (Zondervan 2001). CPP very often leads to extensive medical or even surgical treatment (Howard 2003). Years of disability and suffering are common outcomes (Jaimeson & Steege 1996, Horwitz-Stern & Smolin 2006).

The exact point prevalence of chronic pelvic pain in the female population is not known, but consultations recorded in UK primary care show that the prevalence of CPP was 3.8% in women aged 15–73, a prevalence higher than the prevalence of migraine (2.1%) and almost similar to those of asthma (3.7%) and low back pain (4.1%) (Zondervan et al. 1999, Howard 2003, Warnock & Clayton 2003). Up to 40% of women consulting gynecologists complain of chronic pain in the lower abdomen. Fertile women more often report this type of pain than menopausal women (Zondervan 2001, Grace & Zondervan 2004, Duffy 2001).

It has been estimated that women with chronic pelvic pain use approximately three times more medications of any type than healthy women, and the most commonly used health resource overall was pain medication (Mathias et al. 1996). The resulting costs for health service are considerable, amounting to USD 880 million per year in the US alone (Mathias et al. 1996). The women suffering from CPP present a major challenge to health care, and the lack of treatment success in spite of high costs is frustrating.

Gynecological examination may reveal endometriosis, uterus pathology, ovarian cysts or peri-ovarial peritoneum irritation as the cause of CPP. However, gynecological dysfunction or diseases are frequently not found and about 80% of the patients with chronic pelvic pain have a negative laparoscopy. Thus most authors underscore the need to consider non-gynecological causes of these chronic pain disorders (Slocumb et al. 1984, Beard et al. 1988, Baker 1993, Gunter 2003, Hetrich et al. 2003, Shaeffer 2004, Winkelstein 2004, Jarell 2004). These include disorders that affect the bladder and other parts of the lower urinary tract, diseases of the large bowel, disorders of the lower spine, lumbar plexus, sacrum and pelvis (table 1). Occasionally one of these disorders is present and treatment may be curative. However, even when syndromes or disorders of these organ systems are adequately handled, chronic pain may still persist. Some authors limit the definition of CPP in women to such biomedically unexplained CPP only (Grace 1995; Ehlert & Heim 1999; Bodden-Heidrich et al. 1999, 2001, 2004; Sidentopf & Kentenich 2004; Berberich & Ludwig 2004).

Table 1. Some non-gynecological somatic disorders reported to be associated with CPP

Interstitial cystitis
Chronic relapsing urinary tract infections
Irritable bowel syndrome
Diverticulosis
Inflammatory bowel disease
Neural affection
• Post surgical
• Vertebral disc herniation
• Neoplasms affecting nerve roots or plexa
Joint and/or muscular affection of the sacrum or pelvis

The precise diagnostic classification of biomedically unexplained pain syndromes represent great challenges, as is the case with chronic pelvic pain. Thus, in most cases, CPP will be included in the concept "persistent somatoform pain disorder". International Classification of mental and behavioural Disorders (ICD-10) define such pain as a "persistent severe and distressing pain (which) cannot be explained by evidence of a physiological process or a physical disorder, and the pain is consistently the main focus of the patient's attention"(F.45.4) (WHO 1993, page 108). Accordingly, in CPP no correlation has been found between reported pain and somatic pathology (Ehlert & Heim 1999). However, the pain is exacerbated or occurs in association with emotional distress, conflicts or psychosocial problems (ICD-10 1992, Anonymous, IASP Task on Taxonomy 1994, Sharpe & Carson 2001). By ICD-10 definition, somatoform persistent pain should not occur in the presence of schizophrenia or related disorders, or only during any of the mood disorders; somatization disorder (Briquet's syndrome) or hypo-chondriacal disorder.

If the patient reports other bothersome biomedically unexplained somatic symptoms as well that has lasted for several years and pain is not the dominating symptom—and there is a refusal to accept medical reassurance that there is no adequate physical cause for the physical symptoms—the patient may qualify for the diagnosis undifferentiated somatoform disorder.

In parallel with the concept of alexithymia (the lack of ability to feel or express emotions), women with chronic pelvic pain often lack normal qualities of sensations, exteroceptive as well as proprioceptive (Haugstad 1999, 2000; Kirste et al. 2002). Thus they often lack the ability to be aware of usual somatic sensations, which again leads the patients to exaggerated occupation with the pain that they clearly experience, and further into em-otional states of fear or anxiety related to situations that exacerbates pain. This process may be called "alexisomia" (Kanbara et al. 2004). The patients may thus be characterized by an inability to integrate body sensations with relevant emotions and cognitions, suggesting that dissociative processes also may occur in CPP (Nijenhuis 2004). This lack of normal integration of body awareness and functional cognitive processing may lead the patient into fear for motion (kinesophobia) (Moseley 2003).

Some Aspects of Mechanisms in Longstanding Pain

Pain is a unique experience that is perceived differently by everyone. The spectrum of conceptions of pain may be illustrated by the following two definitions: The first says: "Pain is whatever the experiencing person says it is, existing whenever she says it does" (McCaffery 1968, McCaffery & Pasero 1999, Crooks 2002). This definition acknowledges the uniqueness of pain and makes the patient's self-report the key to pain assessment (Crooks 2002). The other definition of pain used by the International Association for the Study of Pain (IASP) states that: "Pain is an unpleasant sensory and emotional experience associated with actual or potential tissue damage or described in terms of such damage" (Merskey & Bogduk 1994). This definition states the complexity of pain and the existence of both a physical and an emotional component to pain.

Pain can be acute or chronic. Acute pain is usually short-lived and subsides as healing proceeds. The acute pain generally responds well to analgesics, the anatomy and physiology of acute pain is generally well understood and for the most part we are able to manage acute pain effectively (Crook 2002, Gallagher 2005). Chronic pain is generally referred to as lasting longer than 6 months, and may be persisting, intermittent, recurrent or continuous (Breen 2002). In general, antecedent life events, either physical or psychological, seem to change the response to pain, either amplifying or diminishing it. The evaluative or cognitive component is influenced by past experience with pain. Every new episode or change in pain intensity, character or localization activates cognitive processes and emotions that are influenced by the current context and meaning, which are again affected by past pain experiences (Crook 2002, Green 2004, Ursin 2005). In contrast to our ability to manage acute pain, the management of chronic pain often presents a daunting challenge to clinical practice.

In chronic pain the pain threshold is often reduced. The mechanism often referred to, is that signals from the afferent myelinated fibres of the dorsal roots activate spinal neurons normally activated by the thin, unmyelinated nociceptive fibres, second to the plastic changes in spinal and supraspinal structures referred to above, like "memory traces" conveyed by long-term potentiation and similar mechanisms. Minimal stimuli thus lead to the same type of pain that has earlier been associated with painful stimuli. Co-localization of stimuli in space (from anatomical structures adjacent to each other) or time (repeated stimuli) is also conducive of pain formation.

There also seems to be a genetic susceptibility to development of chronic pain syndromes (Kirste et al. 2002). Further, there seems to be an increase in both chronic pain and anxiety in depressed patients, the symptom load increasing with increased severity of depression (Ohayon & Schatzberg 2003; Silverstein 1999, 2002). This phenomenon may be attributed to the influence of input related to affective states (from nuclei known to be involved in emotions like anxiety, i.e., the amygdala) on the sensory "relay stations" such as the thalamus. Such phenomena, often referred to as "gating" of signals, occur at different levels on the signal route from dorsal roots to cortex (Campbell et al. 2003). Sensitization can be understood as an increase in response to a stimulus as function of repeated presentations of that stimulus. Increasing evidence is accumulating in support of the notion that physiological mechanisms of sensitization play an important role in the development of chronic pain syndromes (Russel et al. 1994, Banic et al. 2004).

The lack of an explanation for the causes of the pain can be frightening and frustrating. This can contribute to increased perceived stress and negative interpretations of the symptoms, which in turn may sensitize body and mind (Ursin 1997, Eriksen & Ursin 2002, Lidbeck 2002). Pain behaviour can be considered as a behavioural response to this process. Pain behaviour in chronic pain states is different from the behaviour of acute pain (Breen 2002, Weiner 1999). It can be categorized into expressive behaviours, movement behaviours and functional behaviours. The effects of living with chronic pain adversely alter life patterns resulting in negative physical, psychological, and social effects.

Comorbidity of Chronic Pain

Chronic pain in most instances is associated with other physical or mental symptoms or disorders (such as depression). Psychological modulation of pain is of great importance (Apkarian et al. 2005). For example, negative emotional states have been shown to enhance pain-evoked activity in limbic regions, such as the anterior cingulate and insular cortices (Philips et al. 2003). Further, the anticipation or expectation of pain, activate pain-related areas (see for example Villemure & Bushnell 2002). These facts have led to the development of more complex pain theories. Neuroimaging studies of the human cortical and subcortical physical pain response have identified neural networks consistently referred to as the "pain neuromatrix" (Kelly 2006).

The brain areas that are normally referred to, include the mid/anterior insula, anterior parts of the cingulate cortex, the orbitofrontal cortices and the frontal pole, amygdala and hypothalamus, in addition to the periaqueductal grey matter (Chang 2005, Kulkarni, 2005). It has been hypothesized that activity in the pain inhibition circuits (including those of the corticopontine projections) are reduced when pain is facilitated, together with activation of the limbic and paralimbic circuits (Chang 2005). Kelly et al. (2006) even describe that left caudal anterior cingulate cortex and the left inferior frontal gyrus are activated in persons retrieving autobiographical memories of painful events. Such findings clearly have implications for the understanding of disease mechanisms of chronic pain. Contemporary development in theories of physical therapy and rehabilitation also take these new insights from the neurobiology of pain into consideration in the theoretical frameworks of understanding of chronic pain (Mosely 2003, Tu et al. 2005).

However, additional physical distress symptoms are frequently reported by patients with chronic pain including CPP. Ehlert & Heim (1999) found that CPP patients were suffering from a variety of unexplained bodily symptoms in addition to low abdominal pain, such as vague, diffuse, or overlapping symptoms involving the genitourinary, gastrointestinal, and musculoskeletal systems. They conclude that somatic examinations should not only focus on the predominant pain but also on the additional complaints. Baker (1993), Hetrich et al. (2003), Fitzgerald & Kotarinos (2003) and Tu et al. (2005, 2006) all describe musculoskeletal dysfunction in patients with CPP. Beard (1988) described accumulation of tissue fluids in the hypogastric and inguinal regions. King (1991) described that these patients even had posture and gait disturbances. These findings are corroborated by later studies (Haugstad 2006, Montenegro 2009).

All of this strongly indicates that CPP in most women is a syndrome affecting more than the pelvic area, in particular muscular tension, respiration and functions such as movement and gait. However, despite these reports we are not aware of any study which in a systematic and reliable way has assessed these body functions in women with CPP.

Methods for Assessing Posture, Respiration, Movement Patterns, and Body Awareness

In order to study posture, respiration, movement patterns, and body awareness in women with chronic pelvic pain, the need for a standardized instrument to assess motor functions of the patients and the effect of therapy is apparent. Several instruments to measure motor functions have been developed in the Nordic countries over the course of years. Wilhelm Reich, who stayed in Norway in the 1930s, emphasized the close relationship between repressed emotions and posture, respiration, movements and consistency of muscles (Reich 1968). Following discussions with Reich, the psychiatrist Braatøy and the physiotherapist Bülow-Hansen collaborated to develop the Norwegian psychomotor physiotherapy from the principles formed by Freud and Reich (Bunkan 2001, Bunkan et al. 2002, Bunkan et al. 2003) and also developed a tradition of body examinations.

The most extensive examination is the "Global Physiotherapeutic Muscle Examination" (GPM) developed by Sundsvold and co-workers (1982, 1985). The GPM provides somatic information on the impairment level, and through a scoring system, information about degree of problems (Kvåle et al. 2002, Kvåle et al. 2003a, Kvåle et al. 2003b, Kvåle 2003c, Kvåle et al. 2005). In its most common version it consists of 78 items that cover five main domains: Posture, Respiration, Movement, Muscle and Skin (Kvåle 2003c). It takes a full 45 minutes to perform (Sundsvold et al. 1982, Sundsvold et al. 1985, Kvåle 2003c). Kvåle herself suggest that "a less time-consuming and sounder test battery could be developed, suitable for patients with long-lasting musculoskeletal pain" (Kvåle 2003c). In an effort to simplify this very complex test, Kvåle reduced the test battery from 78 to 52 tests (GPE-52), and was able to demonstrate that this abbreviation could be performed without hampering the reliability or different aspects of the validity (Kvåle et al. 2002, Kvåle 2003c). In spite of this effort to reduce the test size and the amount of time it takes to perform the test, GPE-52 still is quite comprehensive, and takes at best 30 minutes to perform. Moreover, in the GPE-52 test passive elements are dominant, even though it also contains of some active movements performed by the test subject.

Another test battery for body functions likewise developed from the psychomotor physiotherapy tradition, with many features similar to the GPM, is the "Comprehensive Body Examination" (CBE) developed by Bunkan and co-workers (Friis et al. 1998, Bunkan et al. 1999, Bunkan et al. 2001, Bunkan et al. 2002, Friis et al. 2002). Bunkan describes CBE as a refinement of an earlier clinically based body examination (ROBE). Fourteen sub-scales have been developed: two for posture, five for respiration, three for movements and four for muscular consistency (Bunkan 2003). The examination takes about 45 minutes to perform (Bunkan et al. 2002). GPM and CBE are somewhat similar in that they measure ranges of movements and resistance to passive movements in upright and supine positions within a framework of psychodynamic theory formation (Bunkan 2003).

"Body awareness therapy" (BAT) has been independently developed in Sweden (Roxendal 1985). The main aim of this therapy is to integrate the body in the total experience of the self and to restore body awareness and body control (Roxendal 1995). One important aspect of this therapy is the focus on the patient's awareness of sensations and emotions in the body (Gard 2005). This therapy tradition developed the Body Awareness Scale (BAS) to evaluate the effect of the BAT in patients with chronic schizophrenia. The scale has been developed to evaluate the physical as well as the psychic functions of the patient (Bunkan 2003). Roxendal also developed the Body Awareness Scale-Health (BAS-H) [2] (Roxendal 1995, Gyllensten et al. 1999, Gyllensten et al. 2004). The purpose of this scale is to assess patients with psychiatric and psychosomatic diseases, and body empathy in healthy individuals (Roxendal 1985, 1995). The scale (BAS-H) has four main domains (grounding/center line index; centring/breathing index; flow index and additional items index) with a total of 26 sub-indices. The test takes about 30-40 minutes to perform. The BAS-H is strongly connected to a specific theory (the psychodynamic tradition), however, with focus on psychiatric dysfunction. According to

2 BAS-H should be differentiated from Body Awareness Scale which measures somatic arousal (Stegner et al, 1999) and Body Awareness Questionnaire which is an 18-item questionnaire about sensitivity to normal, nonemotive body processes (Shields et al, 1989).

Gyllensten, "Part of the theories of basic BAT and the body ego, defined by Roxendal, are used to analyse the movement function and behaviour with regard to the relation to the ground and the centre line, centring of movements through the movement centre in the solar plexus, freedom of the breathing and the flow of movements throughout the body by the use of the BAS-H" (Gyllensten et al, 2004).

An observer rating scale scoring system called Body Awareness Rating Scale (BARS) was developed by Skatteboe mainly to assess movement harmony, and the purpose was to evaluate the treatment process of Body Awareness Group Therapy for patients with personality disorders (Friis et al. 1989). Twelve items in this scale refer to postural stability, centring, free respireation and mental presence, and this scale is developed from Roxendal's BAS-H.

Other body-oriented treatment methods also exist, like Feldenkrais, Alexander technique, yoga body awareness therapy, etc. (Jain et al. 2004, Schlinger 2006), but these traditions do not include instruments of evaluation of body functions.

This review indicates that there could be a need for a new instrument that can be used to assess the quality of movements according to principles derived from functional anatomy and in keeping with a theoretical framework based on the cognitive abilities of the conscious mental domains. Such an instrument should allow therapists thoroughly trained in observation and visual analysis of the quality of movements to rate the different static and dynamic motor patterns including respiration and gait. In a test based on such dynamic principles, items addressing palpation of muscular consistency and passive movement or handling by the therapist can be excluded. The main focus should be related to active wilful movements performed by the patients as performed in the realm of activities of daily life (Haugstad 2000, Wojniusz 2006). By concentrating on the visual analysis of simple movements, the test should be easy to perform in a clinical setting, only requiring a few minutes, and also be easy to video record for the purposes of training of raters and the evaluation of inter-rater reliability. Thus, we have developed a Standardized Mensendieck Test (SMT) to the end of evaluating posture, movement, gait, sitting posture and respiration and the effect of therapy on these parameters (Haugstad, 2006).

Gynecological Treatment of Chronic Pelvic Pain

Gynecological treatment of chronic pelvic pain may include a variety of measures. Prescription of pain relievers is common, but rarely will medication alone be the solution of chronic pain. Even if there are no symptoms or signs of depression it is also rather common to prescribe antidepressants such as amitriptylin due to their analgetic effects. If the pain has a cyclical pattern, hormone treatments such as birth control pills or other hormonal medications may be prescribed. If an infection is suspected as the source of the pain, antibiotics are used. If tender points are localized, a possible treatment option has also been direct injection of a long-acting local anesthetic into the painful spot (trigger point). In more severe cases nerve ablation or even surgery (intra abdominal tissue ablation, hysterectomy and oophorectomy) has been conducted (e.g., Learman et al. 2007). However, such radical surgical procedure in the absence of localizable pathologies may be challenged, in the want of demonstrable effect, especially when performed at an age below 30 years (Rosenbaum & al., 2008). Most gynecologists also offer different kinds of counselling.

There is a paucity of studies showing clinical improvement of CPP due to these types of intervention (Tu et al. 2005). In a review of all studies on the management of chronic prostatitis / chronic pelvic pain syndrome until 2006, Dimitrakov et al. (2006) similarly concluded that "no universally effective treatment is available that can provide significant lasting benefit for chronic pelvic pain syndrome". Thus women with CPP are often told that no gynecological pathology that may explain their pain has been found (Grace 1995, Duffy 2001) and that no effective treatment is available.

Current Treatment Strategies of Chronic Pain

Since there is an obvious lack of evidence for the effect of traditional gynaecological treatment, it is reasonable to consider treatment studies of chronic pain in general for new treatment options of CPP. There is evidence that cognitive-behavioural therapy applied by interdisciplinary rehabilitation teams may reduce pain in general (Mayou et al. 1997; Lidbeck 1997, 2002; Turk 2003; Baranowski 2009; Wejenborg 2009). Psychological support and cognitive restructuring, explanation of pain mechanism and relaxation techniques often lead to constructive coping and reduced suffering in chronic pain patients (Sharpe 1995, Mayou et al 1997; Lidbeck 1997, 2002; Gullacksen & Lidbeck 2004; Linton 2006). Results obtained from neuro-biological research suggest that cognitive therapy has beneficial biologically demonstrable influences on central pain dysmodulation (Birbaumer et al. 1994, Lidbeck 2002, Gullacksen & Lidbeck 2004). Thus, Mosely (2003) applies the novel insights from functional brain studies of the cerebral neuromatrix of pain in the approach to treatment of patients with chronic pain. Within this model pain is a multiple system output that is activated by an individual-specific pain neuromatrix; activated whenever the brain concludes that body tissue is in danger. The therapeutic aspects of the approach focus on reducing the sensitivity and activity of the pain neuromatrix, via reduction of the perceived threat. The key components are educating the patient in the understanding of pain mechanisms and a systematic approach to desensitizing the pain neuromatrix by gradual increments of the load of motor tasks within the pain limits.

Negative emotional states also contribute to dysfunctional pain modulation mechanisms within the central nervous system (Apkarian et al. 2005, Staud & Domingo 2001), and thus, treatment of these states, like major depression, also could be perceived to improve pain modulation and reduce subjective pain experience. Goldapple et al. (2004) describe how cognitive behavioural therapy alters metabolic rates in the cingulate and frontal cortices. Using imaging techniques, other authors have noticed the effect of distraction on the modulation of pain-evoked activity in the anterior cingulate and insular cortices, as well as in thalamic pain-relaying areas (Apkarian et al. 2005, Hofbauer et al. 2001). Thus, by building both cognitive and motor approaches into the treatment, by changing the focus from pain to other types of sensation from own body, and focusing on coping of simple motor tasks, one would anticipate the activity in pain neuromatrix brain areas become reduced, in parallel with a desensitization to painful stimuli.

Gullacksen and Lidbeck (2004) provided a narrative therapeutic approach. Based on narrative accounts they explained the patient's experience of chronic pain as an understandable process. The authors stated "the individuals who were diagnosed, found the explanation of pain to be a relief and found themselves at the beginning of a whole new process and a long period of healing" (p 151). Once given an explanation of pain (a "pain diagnosis") the patient developed new understanding and gradual improvement of coping skills (Gullacksen & Lidbeck 2004). Several other comprehensive treatment programs of pain also include a strong psychoeducational and cognitive dimension (e.g., Borg-Stein 2006; Osborne et al. 2006; Wigers & Finset 2007).

There are suggestions that a multidisciplinary intervention may be beneficial in the treatment of CPP as well (Rapkin et al. 1987, Kames et al. 1990, Peters et al. 1992, Loeser & Turk 2001, Wesselmann 2001, Greco 2003, Gallagher & Verma 2004, Dick 2004, Gallagher 2005, Wejenborg 2009, Baranowski 2009). Women in group treatment based on psychosomatic and physiotherapeutic principles together with cognitive and behavioural therapy experience reduced pain (Albert 1999). Furthermore, reduction in the use of the National Health Service and increases in gainful employment were registered. Other authors, studying multidisciplinary intervention or physical therapy show pain reduction and better functioning in daily life at end of treatment in patients with CPP (Mattson et al. 2000, Nadler 2002, FitzGerald & Kotarinos 2003, Kotarinos 2003, Anderson et al. 2005, Anderson et al. 2006, Tu et al. 2005, 2008). Randomized controlled intervention studies in this area are, however, quite few.

Physiotherapy as an Integrated Part of Treatment of Chronic Pelvic Pain

In the rehabilitation of patients with chronic pain, physical therapy is often a key aspect of treatment for the achievement of functional restoration. Skilled physiotherapy relies on principles of behavioural medicine (Turk et al. 2000). The therapists use positive reinforcement to instruct, guide, and encourage the patient to engage in physical activities that improve strength, endurance and flexibility (Loeser & Turk 2001). A systematic review found that physical conditioning programs that include a cognitive- behavioural approach plus intensive physical training, given or supervised by physiotherapist or a multidisciplinary team, was efficient in reducing the number of sick days for workers with chronic back and neck pain (Schonstein et al. 2003 a, Schonstein et al. 2003 b).

Both manual physiotherapy and spinal physiotherapy stabilization programs have been reported to be significantly more effective with respect to pain reduction in chronic low back pain patients compared to an active control group (Goldby et al 2006). In other studies of patients with fibromyalgia, physical therapy has also shown positive impact on the patients' general well being, and the patients experienced decreased disability and improved function after physical therapy (Havermark & Lanquis 2006, Wennermer et al. 2006). In musculoskeletal pain disorders several RCT studies have shown promising results in pain and symptom reduction and in self-reported daily functioning improvement (Stuge et al. 2004, Rempel et al. 2006, Maigne et al. 2006, Smeets et al. 2006).

Several studies indicate the effectiveness of similar approaches in other pain conditions as well. In patients with pain related to irritable bowel syndrome (IBS), 12 weeks of basic Body Awareness Therapy (BAT) reduced gastrointestinal and psychological symptoms (Eriksson et al. 2002). Mattson also applied basic BAT as a way of fostering empowerment of women with chronic pelvic pain (CPP), claiming that the women experienced improvement in subjective symptoms after therapy (Mattson et al. 2000). In a non-randomized study of patients with non-specific musculoskeletal disorders, Malmgren-Olsson & Branholm (2002) found larger effect-size in the BAT and Feldenkrais groups compared to regular physiotherapy. However, in a non-randomized study (Kendall et al 2000) of women with fibromyalgia, better results were obtained with a Mensendieck system approach than with BAT. But randomized treatment studies addressing the issue of the most efficient treatment in patients with chronic pain in general or chronic pelvic pain specifically, are lacking.

To summarize, chronic pelvic pain is associated with several non-gynecological symptoms and—as for chronic pain in general—clinical experience and examinations indicate alterations not only in the muscu-loskeletal system, but also increased psychological symptom load. Furthermore, treatment of chronic pelvic pain is extremely difficult and there is a lack of randomized controlled studies showing long-term efficacy. Comprehensive treatment approaches combining physical and cognitive approaches are lacking despite the fact that such treatments seem promising. This suggests that assessments and treatment based on functional anatomy should be of potential efficacy in the treatment of chronic pelvic pain in women. Mensendieck theory and therapy offers this possibility.

Mensendieck Theory and Therapy

Two widely different therapeutic traditions developed from the Paris school of neurology in the early 1900s have made their impact on the development of contemporary physical therapy as well as psychotherapy. Within this outstanding academic center at La Salpêtrière, Duchenne made his groundbreaking studies of neurophysiology (Duchenne, 1872), describing the innervations of muscles, and Charcot taught his students basic and clinical neuropathology. Among their students were Freud, the neurologist who studied hysteric palsies (Freud, 1893) and then went on to formulate his famous theory on the relevance of dreams for understanding the pathology of the subconscious, and Mensendieck, who built explicitly on Duchenne's theories of innervations of muscles of the body, and the central connections all the way up to the primary motor cortex, thus focusing on the cognitive cortical functions of the conscious human, in contrast to the subconscious realm of dreams (Mensendicek, 1937). The roots of dynamic psychotherapy and the later development of psychomotor therapy, that interpret body signs in dynamic categories, are founded on Freud's theories, whereas the later development of cognitive psychotherapy is in keeping with Duchenne's and Mensendieck's focus on the cognitive capacities of the conscious realms of the mind (Beck, 1979). Mensendieck's interest for posture and movements was evident even long before she entered into her medical carrier. She was born American (her maiden name was Elizabeth Varel), married a German, and in the first place went to Paris to study music, singing and sculpturing. While trying to capture and sculpture in stone the appearance of her models, she was struck by their negligent attitude towards own body. She recounts that she asked her teacher why the models had such "floppy bodies". The teacher, apparently perplexed by this comment, replied that she should leave sculpturing in stone, and start sculpturing in flesh and bone (Mensendieck, 1937). This event spurred Bess Mensendieck's medical interest, and she went on to Switzerland to study medicine. Thus, when she later entered the fertile academic environment in Paris, her focus was to sculpture the human body, by virtue of human mind, into something beautiful and also healthy (Mense-ndieck, 1927, Mensendieck, 1954 ("Look better – feel better."). Here she found a perfect instrument in Duchenne's theories.

Mensendieck physiotherapy also contains in germ many of the fundamental principles later developed in theories of motor learning (Fitts et al. 1967; Gentile 1972, 1998; Higgins 1991; Carr et al. 1998; Facchini et al. 2002; Hodges et al. 2002; Flanagan et al. 2003). The focus is on cognitive awareness of experience in own body, and the process of learning new motor patterns in contrast to old habits (Bugge-Rigault 1989, Soukup et al. 1999, Kendall et al. 2000, Haugstad et al. 2000, Kirste et al. 2002, Klemmetsen 2005, Wojniusz 2006). New motor patterns are developed through three phases: 1) the *cognitive* phase, where the conscious awareness of the patient is directed towards sensory input from visual, tactile and proprioceptive stimuli regarding own body, and compared to ideal mentations with regard to the quality of new patterns sought to be obtained; 2) the *associative* phase, where a consciousness gradually develops that integrates the new ideal patterns with new sensory input from the body; and 3) the *automatized* phase, where the new and more efficient or functional motor patterns are utilized without conscious thought, and gradually integrated into behavioral patterns in the activities of daily life. Thus, important basic elements are sensory awareness of own body, conscious cognition of new ideomotor patterns and integrations of the new experience into everyday functions (Mensendieck 1954).

However, it would be a mistake to attribute the application of Mensendieck theory and therapy as it is presented in this study to Bess Mensendieck herself, or to her first line of students. Mensendieck also sought some of her inspiration in the physical fitness program in contemporary Preussian military gymnastics. Thus, even if Mensendieck herself sought to ameliorate the impression of her system of exercises being derived from German military traditions, her later critics have often alluded to this sort of strict upbringing. Mensendieck also never, to our knowledge, herself promoted ideas that would bring her systems of exercises into use within psychiatric care, like Reich, Braatøy and Bülow-Hansen later did with the psychomotor tradition.

The authors were first acquainted with cognitive psychotherapy by Aron Beck's collaborator, Arthur Freeman (1987), when he visited Modum Bad Psychiatric Hospital (Vikersund, Norway) in 1987 as this form of therapy was first introduced into the treatment of anxiety states, in the first place phobic anxiety. It occurred to us that the rigorous and systematic approach to psychotherapy advocated by Freeman and Beck, had strong similarities with the Mensendieck tradition of physiotherapy, as it had been developed over the year in the Oslo school (Halvorsen, 2009). However, a series of amendments had to be made to bring the two therapy traditions into an amalgament. This work was undertaken together with Ulrik Malt at the University of Oslo, in the Department of Psychosomatic Medicine at Rikshospitalet, in the 1990ies. The aim of our work has been to develop instruments to the end of evaluating and treating patients with longstanding pain states and complex disorders, like gynecologic pain, low back pain, chest pain, headache and widespread pain.

The primary goal of the therapy is to develop a good working alliance with the patient, without which therapy would be futile (Lambert et al. 2004). This can be rapidly achieved in the first encounter with the patient, once the therapist opens to empathic listening to the anamnestic history of the patient. The treatment session then can continue by describing a possible explanation for the reported symptoms and a dialogue thus develops between the therapist and the patient with regards to body experiences (see below). The therapist teaches the patients about the mind/body relations, and explaine pain mechanism, in line with the principles of essential cognitive pain education that Lidbeck recommends (2002). Again, the therapist's empathic attitude is of decisive importance to develop the necessary therapeutic alliance with these patients, who often have suffered a lot (Nerdrum 2000 et al., Nerdrum 2002, Hersoug 2002).

Mensendieck therapists are trained to assess motor function both in terms of global quality of movement and in the detailed function of every muscle group in the body (Mensendieck 1937, 1954; Haugstad et al. 2000; Kirste et al. 2002; Klemmetsen 2005). Thus, it can be said that the Mensendieck tradition is founded on the principles of functional anatomy. However, Bess Mensendieck was also deeply aware of the fact that the generation of movements is a mental task, and that this task could be brought to conscious attention by mentally rehearsing the movement ahead of time, before the physical execution of the movement proper. Thus, the training programs start with the "teacher" and "pupil" imagining ("sketching") the movement to be practiced (Mensendieck, 1927, 1937, 1954). In physiologic terms, this preparation for movement involves several areas frontal to the primary motor cortex (Facchini et al. 2002, Flanagan et al. 2003, Andersen 2003). This form of ideomotor preparation of the movement proper, called "motor templates", have been shown to enhance motor learning (Fitts 1954, Faccini et al. 2002, Flanagan et al. 2003). The focus on the cognition preceding movement, as well as the focus on practicing new motor patterns in the activities of daily life, can also be said to be more in keeping with cognitive therapy, developed by Ellis, Beck, Freeman and others (Beck 1976, Freeman 1987, Reinecke 1996).

An additional important aspect of Mensendieck therapy is focus on the state of tension of a specific group of muscles or agonist. The patient's awareness is guided towards increase of tension in the muscle (maximal contraction), and the decrease of tension (maximal relaxation). This awareness of tension and relaxation is also sought to be automatized into the movements of daily living, much in keeping with the principles of "applied relaxation" (Öst 1987).

Similar to patients in cognitive therapy, the patients treated by a Mensendieck therapist are always assigned graded tasks to be practiced several times each day, preferably while performing the activities of a normal life (Mensendieck 1927, 1954). Thus, the new motor programs are sought to be automatized and internalized in the patient including the pattern of tension and relaxation of agonist and antagonist muscle groups. Further, the Mensendieck physiotherapy trainees are taught in a systematic way to be aware of own bodily experience, thus developing a high level of body awareness themselves, an awareness always sought to be transferred to the "pupil" or the "patient" (Mensendieck 1954, Rigault 1989, Soukop 1999, Haugstad 2000, Kendall et al. 2000, Klemmetsen 2005, Haugstad et al.2006).

The mental aspects of the effort it takes to change ingrained motor patterns are sometimes underestimated. In the Mensendieck tradition, this focus has been quite clear from the original works of Bess Mensendieck. However, the mental parts of therapy may at some points in time have caught less attention than the biomechanical and anatomical aspects of the tradition. In our opinion, it is the integration of mind and body that are so characteristic of this tradition within physical therapy. And it is this integrative approach that we have sought to bring to attention in our work within the field of psychosomatic medicine. Thus, to underline the cognitive aspect of Mensendieck therapy and remind the reader to keep the mental aspects of the therapeutic approach in conscious attention, we prefer the term "somatocognitive therapy"[3] as label of the treatment approach that we apply in this study.

Somatocognitive Therapy

Somatocognitive therapy can thus be understood as a hybrid between physiotherapy and psychotherapy. As such, it is a short-term body-oriented therapy, concentrating on the situation here and now—not focusing on the possible historical roots of the symptoms. The goal is to achieve new body awareness through explorative treatment with functional goals linked into the activities of daily living. As sessions evolve, the therapy necessarily leads to the disclosure of repressed emotions. This is not the primary goal of the therapy, but on the other hand, emotions should be given room and be received by the empathic therapist. The therapist and the patients are seen as equally important partners in exploring the experiences of the patient. Like in cognitive therapy, the therapy session is three-phased: 1) The patient recounts from his or her experience since the last session, reports on homework done, and possible new experiences or insights evolved through the new movements

[3] The concept "somatocognitive" in this setting refers to the therapeutic approach combining a somatic and cognitive approach and should not be confused with the "somatocognitive theory of emotion" proposed by Schachter (Schachter & Singer 1962). This theory is based on attribution research where emotions are interpreted as a result of (unspecific) neurovegetative excitation (arousal) and certain characteristics of the external situation (the so-called cognitions).

that have been practiced in the activities of daily living. 2) Learning new active movements in a graded task assignment—again to be practiced several times each day, not as separate exercise sessions, but well integrated in the activities of the day, like while walking to the bus, sitting in the office, lying down in bed, watching the television, while eating, performing house chores, etc. This may influence muscle relaxation, respiration, the flexibility of joints, muscles and ligaments, straining work loads on muscles and joints, extero- and proprioception, awareness of own body, and reduced fear for movements (kinesophobia). It is of utmost importance that the training is started in a gentle manner, and that exercise is not exceeding the patient's capacities in any way. These patients have often a long story of suffering from aches and pains, which involve them in a passive lifestyle with fear for movement. An abrupt change to vigorous physical activity may result in physiological responses characterized by increased pain, due to mechanisms like long term potentiation (LTP) and wind-up (Staud, 2005). Often manual release of the tensed muscles may be given, with a dual purpose: First, it improves the circulation of the relevant muscle and leads to new tactile experiences, and secondly, it leads to release of endogenic substances like oxytocin (Meyer-Lidenberg, 2008), that are known to promote relaxation and foster bonding between therapist and patient. The second part of the therapy session is always concluded with a brief session of applied relaxation. 3) New assignments are given for the homework of the patient, again underscoring that the most important part of therapy takes place during the intervals between therapy sessions. The therapist constantly assures that the patient understands the significance of each step, and that the working alliance is upheld.

Application of Somatocognitive Therapy in a Clinical Setting: A Randomized, Controlled Intervention Study

In a recent study, we sought to apply the principles described above in an intervention study with women with CPP. The main aims of this study were to study the complex motor patterns of posture, movement and coordination, gait, sitting posture and respiration, and to study the effect of somatocognitive therapy on these and other outcome variables. As part of this effort, the aim was also to develop and evaluation instrument specifically designed to assess these complex motor functions.

Materials and Methods

CPP Patients, Inclusion and Exclusion Criteria

During the period 1998–2003 women between 20 and 50 years with pelvic pain duration between 1 and 10 years referred to the outpatient department of gynecology in a tertiary care university hospital (Rikshospitalet, The National Hospital, Oslo, Norway), were consecutively considered suitable for inclusion in our study. A full medical record and clinical examination was obtained, including a gynecological examination and palpation of the pelvic muscles, and a thorough history of pain. Patients were excluded from the study if there was evidence of somatic diseases such as multiple sclerosis, stenosis of the lumbar spinal canal or traumatic damage of the spinal cord/cone/spinal roots or nerves, lumbar disc herniation, pelvic instability, cancer, Mb. Crohn, ulcerating colitis, trapped ovary syndrome or pain localized to the vulvae only.

Table 2. Inclusion and exclusion criteria for the selection of patients to the randomized, controlled intervention study involving women with chronic pelvic pain

Inclusion criteria	Exclusion criteria
Women	Somatic disease
20-50 years	Pain in vulva only
Chronic pelvic pain	Psychiatic exlusion criteria; serious personality disorder lifetime psychosis organic brain disease major depression serious anorexia or bulimia
Pain duration 1-10 y	
	Pelvic instability
	Lumbar root affection

Secondly the patients were examined by a clinical psychologist at the Department of Neuropsychiatry and Psychosomatic Medicine at Rikshospitalet that performed a standard psychological interview and examination, including psychometric evaluation. The psychiatric exclusion criteria were the following: serious personality disorder, lifetime psychosis, bipolar disorder, organic brain disease, major depression, drug or alcohol dependency, and serious anorexia or bulimia.

Finally, the patients were examined by a Mensendieck physical therapist with a full standard clinical examination, including Lasegue's test to exclude lumbar nerve root affection, and pelvic examination to exclude pelvic instability (see *table 2*).

Key functions assessed by the Standardized Mensendieck Test Optimal score 7, poorest score 0	
Posture	Score
Global/line of gravity	
Ankle	
Knee	
Pelvis	
Back	
Shoulder	
Neck	
Average	
Gait	Score
Global	
Foot roll	
Propolsion	
Rotation	
Average	
Movement	Score
Global	
Frontal armlift	
Vertical armlift	
Sagital armswing	
Diagonal armswing	
Balance/hip flexion	
Average	
Sitting posture	Score
Global	
Support	
Pelvis	
Back	
Average	
Respiration	Score
Global	
Armlift	
Pelvic lift	
Average	

Figure 1. The women included in the study were scored for motor patterns with regards to posture, movement, gait, sitting posture and respiration. See Methods for explanation. For further details, see Haugstad et al., (2006 a, appendix).

DEVELOPMENT OF A STANDARDIZED MENSENDIECK TEST (SMT)

A standardized Mensendieck Test (SMT) was developed to evaluate posture, movement, gait, sitting posture, and respiration of patients with chronic pelvic pain, based on the Mensendieck principles of observation and analysis of motor function (Figure 1). To validate the test and to make a comprehensive body examination of a defined group of patients, it was applied in this study of women with chronic pelvic pain (Haugstad 2000).

The first 15 patients who fulfilled the inclusion criteria (women averaged 32.3 years (SEM 1.43) were compared with 15 matched healthy controls using the SMT test for examination of motor function. These 15 healthy women were almost in the same age range (mean age 30 y, range 22–50 y), and educational background, randomly recruited from students and employees at the Oslo College and The National Hospital. All the 30 women were videotaped when they performed the Standardized Mensendieck Test, and three Mensendieck physiotherapists examined the video to validate the test. Raters had no information about the status of the subjects. Each element of the test was assigned a score from 0 to 7, where 0 is the least functional movement, and 7 the score for an optimal performance.

THE CHARACTERISTICS OF PATIENTS WITH CPP

To describe the body characteristics of the patients with CPP we included 40 + another 20 women having fulfilled the above-mentioned criteria. The additional 20 patients were recruited in the same way as described above. All were clinical interviewed by the physiotherapist. The 15 healthy female matched controls are described above. All the patients and the healthy control women were examined by The Standardized Mensendieck test (SMT). The examination was video recorded. For the 60 chronic pelvic pain patients a visual analogue score of pain (VAS) was obtained. In order to obtain a more thorough evaluation of muscle function, we also examined several muscle groups for elasticity and density and for subjective experience of pain, in addition to the SMT and the VAS score. The muscle was said to have normal, high, or very high density and elastic stiffness, scored as 0 for normal, 1 for high and 2 for very high. The subjective experience of pain in the muscles under the palpation was also marked with 1 for painful and 2 for very painful.

The muscles that were systematically examined were femoral adductor muscles, the iliopsoas muscles, the abdominal muscles, the muscles in the gluteal region and outward rotators of the hip.

THE RANDOMIZED CONTROLLED INTERVENTION STUDY AND THE 1 YEAR FOLLOW-UP STUDY

Having fulfilled the inclusion criteria, the patients were recruited to the intervention study, and the standardized Mensendieck test performed and recorded on video tapes (v.i.). 40 patients with chronic pelvic pain were randomized into the two treatment groups: 1) Standard gynecological treatment (STGT) and 2) STGT + Mensendieck somatocognitive therapy (MCST). The treatment period was 3 months (90 days). Group 1 received standard gynecological advice at inclusion and one more time during the treatment period. Group 2 received 10 treatments sessions with the Mense-ndieck therapist of 1 hour's duration over 90 days. The randomization occurred by drawing a folded piece of paper with the patient's name from a jar, thus allocating the name to a previously chosen treatment group. The randomization was performed by a person external to the study. At the time when the patients were randomized into the treatment groups, a visual analogue score of pain (VAS) (Jensen et al. 1986, Strong et al. 2002) was obtained. They were asked to assess, each day during the first week of the study, their subjective experience of pain on a scale from 0 to 10, and mark the score on a straight line, 0 to the left and 10 to the right, with 0 denoting no pain, and 10 a maximum of pain experience. The average of the daily scores for this week was taken as baseline value.

After the treatment period was completed, a new gynecological, psychological/ psychometric and Mensendieck examination was conducted, including a second video recording of the patients performing the Standardized Mensendieck Test (SMT). These video tests were blinded so that the evaluator did not know whether the patients on the video were in the control group or in the treatment group. The same VAS scores procedures was also performed. One year after inclusion the same examinations were done for the third time for all the patients.

Psychological Assessments

Visual analogue scales are frequently used ways of measuring an individual's perception of specific phenomena or symptoms such as pain or distress. However, VAS scales do not have predefined severity steps. Thus each individual uses the VAS with their own internal reference for severity in mind. This procedure explains why VASs are valid and sensitive assessments tools from an individual perspective. The drawback, however, is limited validity when comparing group data. For this purpose, rating scales, symptom checklists or questionnaires are more suitable. They provide the patient with pre-defined categories (e.g. a little bit, some; much; very much or less than usual; as usual; more than usual). For example: a VAS score of 70 (0-100) on a distress scale may by one person be labelled "much", by another "very much". This difference in evaluation of the severity of the symptom will be detected by the questionnaire, but not by the VAS score. This well-known fact indicates that when evaluating treatment outcome both VASs and questionnaires with predefined severity or frequency steps should be employed for optimal description.

During the last thirty years, a large amount of self-rating scales, checklists and questionnaires have been published addressing phenomena such as quality of life, distress, psychosomatic symptoms, social and occupational function. In our study we decided that besides pain, two major classes of phenomena were crucial targets for treatment: inability to continue to carry out one's normal "healthy" functions, and the appearance of new phenomena of a distressing nature. Thus we wanted a questionnaire that addressed these two phenomena and which was sensitive to change. Secondly, we wanted to use a scale that was well-validated and widely used in different medical and psychosomatic populations including pain and gynaecology. The General Health Questionnaire (GHQ) meets all these requirements (Goldberg & Williams 1988).

Huppert and co-workers (1989) factor analyzed the GHQ-30 and found five factors: (1) anxiety and insomnia; (2) depression; (3) general well-being; (4) social function and (5) coping. The anxiety sub-scale (8 items) includes symptoms of worrying, inner tension, self confidence and general distress. The focus is on cognitive aspects of anxiety. The depression sub-scale (5 items) addresses a more clinical dimension of depression with questions on guilt, pessimistic thoughts, lassitude and suicidal ideation. The well-being sub-scale (4 items) addresses issues such as vitality, well-being and life satisfaction. The coping subscale (5 items) covers adaptation and self-assertiveness. The social dysfunction scale only has 3 items dealing with relation to and content with relationships to other persons.

RESULTS

Intraclass Correlation among the Raters in Evaluation of the SMT

The $ICC_{1.1.}$ values ranged between 0.83 (subscore for the position of the back) to 0.97 (several subscores for movement; gait and sitting posture). The SMT showed good discriminative ability when examining these two groups. Patients with CPP scored significantly lower than the controls on every subtest. In particular, scores were low for movement (coordination), gait (rotation of the pelvis relative to the spinal column) and for respiration (respiratory response on pelvic lift). The values ranged between 0.83 (posture, subscores for position of the back, 95 % C.I. between 0.63 and 0.92) and 0.97 (respiration) in the evaluation among the raters. The power of the Mensendieck assessment technique to discriminate between patients with CPP and the controls was calculated and the sensitivity and specificity of the test was good to excellent. Despite the fact that the testing was blinded with regard to the the test subjects status, we found that the agreement among the testers was generally better when assessing patients than when assessing the healthy controls.

Clinical Characteristics of CPP Patients

The average score for the subjective pain (VAS) for all 60 patients was 6.01 (SD ± 1.51; SEM ± 0.21; range 3-8), on a scale from 0 to 10.75% of the patients had moderate or severe pain during or after intercourse. 50% of the patients described this as aching in one or both inguinal regions and also in the sub umbilical region. 25% reported that pain started after infection in the bladder or kidney region, and 25% told that the pain developed after an abortion or after a hard labour. 15–20% had a recount of sexual abuse. They experienced their whole body as painful, with no pleasurable sensations left. They also reported lack of contact and control with whole regions of their bodies.

Posture and Movement Patterns Assessed with the SMT

All subscores found in the patients were significantly lower (p levels < 0.01) than those of the healthy controls. The largest difference in scores between the two groups was found for gait, movement and respiration. The subscores were 54% lower for pelvic rotation in the gait group of scores and 52% lower for pelvic lift in the respiration group and diagonal arm swing in the movement group, respectively, compare with the healthy controls. The least difference between the patients and the controls were found in the subscores for posture. The greatest deviation from normal pattern was found for tests that posed a demand on balance and coordination. In the test for hip flexion, the patients had great difficulties when trying to stand on one leg for 10 seconds, scoring 38% below the healthy controls. Further, their ability to coordinate the movements of both arms and both legs in the sagital (33%) and diagonal arm swing tests (39%) were well below the healthy controls. The ability to give in to gravity was found to be reduced for the patients compared to controls, when testing their ability to lift extended arms to shoulder height, and let them fall down. When examinating gait we observed a careful gait with short steps and almost no foot propulsion, and a markedly reduced hip extension in the propulsion phase. The typical findings in respiration are high costal respiration with almost no movement in the thorax or in the abdominal area (Haugstad, 2006a, appendix). In the evaluation of respiration the scores differed 52% from the healthy women. The movement pattern may be ascribed to what we call a typical pelvic- pain- protection pattern (ppp). The patients protect their pelvic in gait, movement and in the respiration.

Findings in Muscle Palpation

Highest density and highest degree of elastic stiffness were found in the following muscles: iliopsoas in density and 1.59 ± 0.09 in elastic stiffness. Iliopsoas was also most painful 1.60 ± 0.09. Almost the same scores were found in the straight abdominal muscles with 1.52 ± 0.10 in density, 1.53 ± 0.10 in elastic stiffness and 1.53 ± 0.10 in tenderness. The femoral adductors also had high scores; 1.41 ± 0.11 (density) and 1.38 ± 0.11 (elastic stiffness and tenderness).

The Effect of the Mensendieck Somatocognitive Therapy

The Effect of Treatment after Three Months

After 90 days of treatment the CPP patients in the Mensendieck somatocognitive therapy group (MSCT) had significantly improved scores in all subtests of the SMT. The patients receiving standard gynecological treatment only (STGT) for the most part did not show any significant changes of scores. The best treatment response in the STGT + MSCT group was found in the case of scores for respiration. The second group of functions that improved considerably was in the subtests for movement. The patients demonstrated the largest improvement in the movement tests functions designed to demonstrate coordination, and the ability to relax. The average SMT score values after treatment were 4.37 ± 0.38 (up 19.3%) for posture, 4.13 ± 0.38 (up 26.1%) for movement, 4.13 ± 0.39 (up 24.8%) for gait, 4.67 ± 0.36 (up 27.9%) for sitting posture, and a considerable increase to 4.72 ± 0.37 (up 58.4%) in the scores for respiration.

The patients' subjective experience of pain was assessed by means of a visual analogue (VAS) pain scale. Before treatment, the patients were randomized into the group receiving standard gynecological treatment scored an average of 6.68 ± 0.29 (average ± standard error). After the treatment period of 90 days, the average VAS score was 6.16 ± 0.50, a reduction by 7.8 % (non-significant). The patients in the Mensendieck somatocognitive therapy group scored an average of 5.60 ± 0.40 at baseline. After the 90 days' treatment program, the average score was 2.89 ± 0.40, down by 48.4 %. This corresponds to an effect size of 1.5 and a number needed to treat (NNT) of 1.9, both based on the VAS scores.

Effect after One Year Follow Up

When the patients were evaluated with a new SMT and VAS nine months after end of treatment, the patients in the group receiving standard gynecological treatment showed no significant change in motor performance. At one year follow up, the tendencies for the performance of the motor functions on a general level was an increased deterioration, even significantly for some of the subtests in the STGT group.

By contrast, the patients receiving Mensendieck somatocognitive therapy demonstrated improved scores after treatment. Moreover the effect of therapy lasted for the 9 months follow-up period and for most functions even improved further after end of therapy. The scores nine months after treatment month were 4.66 ± 0.30 (up 4.0 %, non significant change from end of treatment) for posture, 4.85 ± 0.33 (up 13.0 %, $p < 0.02$) for movement, 4.54 ± 0.39 (up 10.0 %, $p < 0.001$) for gait, 5.01 ± 0.36 (up 7.2%, non-significant change from end of treatment) for sitting posture, and a considerable increase to 5.36 ± 0.35 (up 13.5%, $p < 0.05$) in the scores for respiration.

The largest change nine months after treatment was seen in the respiratory response to the lifting and lowering the arms from the supine position ("armlift" see the test manual, appendix of Haugstad et al., 2006a). Score for this function increased from 4.68 ± 0.31 to 5.50 ± 0.39 (up 20.2%, $p < 0.01$). Further, the improvement was greatest for the subscales for rotation in gait, and diagonal arm swing and hip flexion in movement.

The patients' subjective experience of pain was assessed by means of a visual analogue (VAS) pain scale. Nine months after treatment the average pain was 6.13 ± 0.39, a reduction by 0,5 % from 90 days (non-significant). In contrast the patients in the Mensendieck treatment group scored an average of 2.21 (± 0.44) at nine months compared to 5.60 ± 0.40 at baseline and 2.89 ± 0.40 after 90 days of treatment. Thus there is a further significant reduction from 3 to 9 months in the treatment group ($p < 0.003$). NNT was 2.9, and effect size 1.0.

The mean case and likert scores were relatively low at inclusion for the STGT and MSCT groups respectively (5.19 and 28.19 versus 7.61 and 31.33). Nevertheless there was a statistical significant decrease in sub-scale scores for coping and anxiety-insomnia-distress in the MSCT-group, but not in the STGT group only. The reduction in the subscale for depressive symptoms (from 3.39 to 2.62) was almost statistical significant in the MSCT-group ($p=0.06$), but not for the STGT group where an increase occurred (2.13 to 2.92; $p=0.17$). However, when only looking at the GHQ-30 likert total score the reduced in the MSCT-group from 31.33 to 26.54 was not statistical significant ($p=0.12$). There was a non-significant increase in total likert score in the STGT-group (from 28.19 tol 30.15; $p=0.28$).

The NNT and effect size based on GHQ-total likert scores were 4.3 and 0.7, respectively. The coping and anxiety-insomnia subscales showed NNT and effect size scores of 3.2/1.2 and 3.2/0.6, respectively. The NNT values are calculated from a treatment effect of at least 50 %.

DISCUSSION

The main aim of this study was *a)* to develop a better understanding and more knowledge of women with chronic pelvic pain, including a body oriented treatment approach, and to apply this treatment in a randomized controlled treatment study, including the mental elements of recognizing body function, concentrating on motor expressions and learning of new patterns (somatocognitive therapy). As part of this aim, we wanted to *b)* develop an evaluation instrument specifically designed to describe complex motor patterns of posture, movements and coordination, gait, sitting posture and respiration (the SMT test).

The Standardized Mensendieck Test

The test discriminated well between women with chronic pelvic pain and matched healthy women.

With respect to the overall validity of the test, it should be noted that there are three principal ways of establishing validity (American Psychological Association, 1974): 1) content validity (demonstrating that the test samples the proper domain of items), 2) criterion-related validity (demonstrating that scores of the test correlate with other independent measures that are called criteria) and 3) construct validity (showing that hypotheses derived from theory are confirmed when tested by empirical research; Schontz 1986). We have demonstrated that the SMT test samples relevant data (i.e., it shows *content validity*), that the test demonstrates significant differences between groups defined by different criteria like healthy women and women with CPP (i.e., it shows *criterion-related validity*), and that it demonstrates that the hypothesized deviation from normal motor patterns of the CPP patients are indeed found to be deviant when applying the test (i.e., it shows *construct validity*).

We have concluded that the SMT showed good *discriminative validity*. Thus it should be understood that we hereby refer to the finding that the test discriminated well between CPP patients and healthy controls.

Several explanations can be proposed. One may question whether the evaluating physical therapist was really "blinded", i.e., whether some bias could still come into play. CPP patients have a characteristic pain behaviour that easily can be spotted by the evaluator. For example, some of the patients could not walk without a stick, others could not lift their arms because of the stretch in the abdomen, and some could not stand on one leg without holding on to something. This problem would generally apply to any study of patients that have altered behaviour or motor patterns, and is thus not a specific problem of this particular study. Still, it cannot be excluded that a bias stemming from these differences in patients' appearance could have influenced the rating of patients, thus providing less variance of scores. However, the greater variability in the scoring of the controls may reflect difference in the opinion among the therapists as to what pattern of movement is perceived to be optimal or "normal". On the other hand, when patients were assessed by the SMT, the agreement among the evaluators was generally good, with excellent agreement in evaluating the pattern of movement, gait and respiration. This may indicate that the patients with CPP display a stereotypical pattern of movement dysfunction that is clearly perceived to deviate from normal variation. The deviations from normal patterns were most clearly demonstrated in the tests for movement, gait and respiration.

This corresponds to others studies using different assessments. The GPE-52 domains Respiration and Movement also showed higher ICC scores in patient groups in the Kvåle study (2003). Thus it is likely that experienced physiotherapists observe deviations from normal patterns in patients with chronic muscle pain, and most clearly so in the tests for movement and respiration.

Based on SMT alone, it would be possible to discriminate between women with CPP and asymptomatic women. However, this does not imply that the SMT would suffice as tool to categorize a woman as having pelvic pain, because no comparison has been made with patients with other psychosomatic or psychiatric symptoms. In the future we have to use the SMT to validate the test on different patient groups other than CPP.

The Effect of Somatocognitive Treatment

Methodological Considerations

In our randomized material, the women of the two treatment groups are similar with regard to average age, number of labors, depression scores and the frequency of dyspareunia, irritable bowel syndrome and muscle and joint pains (Haugstad et al., 2006c). However, in spite of the blinded randomization procedure there were slight differences with regard to educational level and the subjective pain level in the two groups. In the STGT group none of the women had college education; in the MSCT group 7 of the patients had education from college. Still, when college and high school education were seen together, 12 women in the each group had higher level education. Thus, overall the educational level may be said to be reasonably equal in the two groups.

In the two treatment groups the baseline VAS scores were also a bit different. The VAS average score in the STGT group was 6.68 (± 0.29), one point higher than in the MSCT group (5.60 ± 0.40). After 3 months treatment the VAS score reduction in the MSCT group was great almost 50% down (2.89 ± 0.40) compare to the STGT group reduction after 3 months that was only 7.8 % (non significant). We have no good explanation for this differences in baseline VAS score in the two groups, other than that they are probably within the range that could be explained by random variation in two groups of 20 CPP patients.

Possible Mechanisms behind the Improvement in SMT and VAS Scores after Somatocognitive Treatment

In the very beginning of the somatocognitive therapy the patients and the therapist have to establish a good therapeutic alliance. The empathic therapeutical attitude is of great importance for the outcome of the treatment in all types of therapies (Gyllensten et al. 1999, Hersoug 2001, Hoffart et al. 2002, Nerdrum & Rønnestad 2003, Ekerholt & Bergland 2004, Ryum & Stiles 2005). In the past decade, the working alliance has emerged as possibly the most important conceptualization of the common elements in diverse therapy modalities. The working alliance is the product of the patient's and the therapist's conscious determination and ability to work together. No successful therapy can take place without a working alliance which is equivalent to a working relationship in any team effort outside the therapeutic setting (Hersoug 2001, Nerdrum & Rønnestad 2003).

A good working alliance requires that the patient is able to look at himself objectively together with the therapist. It is seen as a prerequisite that the patient perceives the therapist to have a supportive attitude. Thus trust and belief the therapist's abilities and genuine motivation to help are invaluable assets in the therapeutic setting. The therapeutic working alliance has been shown to be of importance for the outcome of the therapy, and Hersoug

(2001), concludes that patients prefer therapists that are actively involved in treatment and treatment planning.

It is necessary to have achievable functional goals for the treatment. Examples of such goals from our study could be “to learn breathing more deeply”, ”learn walking without a stick”, ”sleep in the prone position”, ”sit on both tuber ischii”, “touch the abdomen” and “try to have sex again”. In line with cognitive therapy the somatocognitive therapy formulate an agenda for every session. Typical agenda items might include a review of the week (brief, and focused on items of relevance), review of the homework, particular items to be worked on within the session and how to practice the learned techniques (Freeman et al. 1987, Beck et al. 1979). The final few minutes of the session can be used to evaluate the session, go over homework for the next session, and have the patient encapsulate what she has learned during the session and will be taking home with her. An aspect of great significance in both somatocognitive and cognitive therapy is the idea that the therapy does not happen 1 or 2 hours a week in the therapist’s office, but needs to be a process that is constantly lived. An important part of the collaboration is for the patient to do the self-help work at home, in daily life. Clinical experience has indicated that the patients who do more self-help work make progress more quickly in therapy and are able to meet their stated therapy goals more rapidly (Freeman et al. 1986).

A word of caution should be added when discussing the different outcomes of the two treatment groups. The frequency of therapeutic sessions was clearly different in the two groups. Where as the women in the STGT group had all together 7 visits to the therapists during the 10 weeks’ intervention period, the women in the MSCT group had all together 7 + 10, i.e. 17 visits to the therapists, a considerably larger number of consultations. 10 of these sessions were with one of the therapists, the Mensendieck therapist. Thus, the possibility that the empathic alliance formed by this latter therapist in itself, or the positive expectations formed by the knowledge that this intervention was perceived to be a new and exciting procedure by the whole team could explain the favorable outcome in these women, independent of the specific therapeutic procedures, can not be entirely ruled out. The strength of evidence that MSCT itself works, would be increased if future studies can be performed with equal numbers of consultations in the STGT and STGT + MSCT groups.

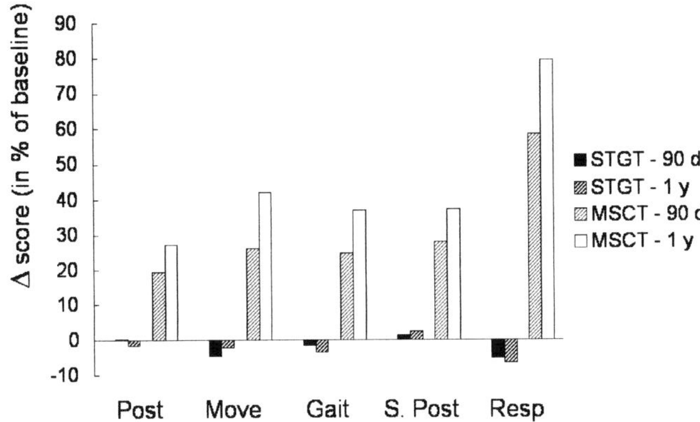

Figure 2. The figure shows change in scores, in % of baseline before therapy, for motor pattern after therapy and at one years follow-up (for posture, movement, gait, sitting posture and respiration, for standard gynaecological treatment black and densely hatched bars, for somatocognitive therapy, lightly hatched and open bars.

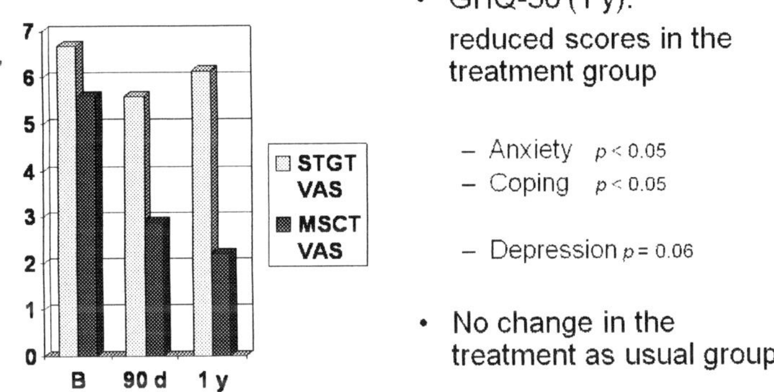

Figure 3. To the left, the light bars show the VAS pain scores for control patients (B = baseline, 90 day = after therapy and 1 year = at follow-up), whereas the dark bars show the VAS score for the patients subjected to somatocognitive therapy at the same points in time. To the right, the level of statistical significance for change in mental distress after therapy as measured by the general health questionnaire (GHQ-30) instrument.

Respiration

In this study the pattern of respiration is the subtest in the SMT where the patients improve the most during the 90 days of Mensendieck somatocognitive therapy. In Mensendieck therapy there is always a focus on a functional respiration (Mensendieck 1954, Haugstad 1999, 2000). The patients are taught how to fill the lung so the thoracic rib cage and abdomen move. In the initial sessions the patients should register their breathing pattern and how they could change the breathing to more functional and freer respiration. They learnt this through new movements and cognition, (Mensendieck Exercises, Klemmetsen 2004), through pedagogical instructions and through careful manual release ("sykegrep") of tender musculature around the abdomen and in the pelvic area (Lingsten & Halvorsen 2001). The patients were assigned homework between sessions, i.e. breathing lessons to be performed during daily activities; when they sit watching TV, relax on the sofa, or work on the PC. It was found typical for the patients in the study to state that they "had not dared to breathe down in the abdomen because of the pain". In somatocognitive therapy we start changing the focus, from pain experiences in the body to experiences of new movements in daily life. It was seldom for the patients to experience these new movements as scaring or unpleasant. This strategy of "changing the focus" is an important element in the patient's path out of the vicious circle of negative thoughts and actions. This can be seen to be in line with a theory of "desensitization" (Mosely 2003).

Movement

The second group of functions that improved considerably after somatocognitive therapy was the subtests for movements. The patients demonstrated the largest improvement in the tests functions designed to demonstrate coordination and the ability to relax. Other authors have also demonstrated that there seem to be a relationship between the experience of pain and the ability to relax as well as other aspects of motor functions (Kvåle 2003, Kvåle et al. 2005). In this study we found an altered pattern of movements and "no touching" of hypersensitive and swollen abdominal area. We have ascribed the term a "pelvic pain protecting pattern" this particular cluster of behaviours. The typical pattern described (Haugstad et al., 2006b) correlates to the well-known "guarded behaviour" in patients with low back pain, which may either be due to the pain itself or to the fear of pain (Hamaoui et al. 2002, Lamoth et al 2003, Vlayen et al. 2007). The Mensendieck somatocognitive therapy starts the therapy with the simplest forms of movements that may be used in daily life, moving to the more complex exercises when the simple ones are automatized. New baselines are created (Moseley 2003). This learning of movement is well known from neuropsychology and from sport sciences (Fitts et al. 1964, Gentile 1998, Hodges & Franks 2002). The new movements will focus on normal use of the muscles, and focus on the movement itself, without paying attention to the pain. Mensendieck somatocognitive therapy also include the element of manual release of tender muscles in the pelvic region, in keeping with the approach physical therapy traditions in general, as demonstrated in other studies (Fitzgerald et al. 2003, 2005, Kotarinos et al. 2003, Anderson et al. 2005, 2006, Cornel et al. 2005). The various manual techniques and modalities could open up for more free movements and more functional use of the muscles both in gait and in coordination of movements.

Pain

Mensendieck somatocognitive treatment changed the level of experienced pain for the CPP patients with an average of almost 50 % in VAS score. Seven of the 20 patients in the treatment group were quite pain free after treatment (VAS 0-2), they respond very well to the MSCT. Two of the patients in the MSCT group had not responded specifically to the treatment and the pain was almost same in intensity after treatment (VAS 6-7). These two patients were not responding well enough to this treatment (Haugstad et al., 2006c). The others had significantly reduction in pain after three months with MSCT. With regard to possible mechanisms involved in the pain reduction, we suggest that the reasons might be more functional movement, changes in gait, improved posture with more relaxed pattern, reduction in fear for movements etc. All of these changes would imply a change of focus from pain experience to positive body experiences and coping of daily activities. According to the pain neuromatrix theory, these changes would occur simultaneously with reduced brain activity in the correspondeing areas, i.e. anterior cingulate and insular cortices. In addition, we have observed less swelling of the lower abdomen and inguinal areas, implying improved lymphatic drainage through better circulation. With respect to the positive development in body awareness in these women, we would like to emphasize the importance of the ideomotor preparation for the movement proper. Mensendieck training is focusing on the mental ideation of movements, thus increasing the patient's conscious awareness of both proprioceptive and exteroceptive sensory input. We tend to believe that this carefully developed method of patient instruction is a prerequisite for the relatively rapid improvement in the patient's acquaintance with her own body. With regards to the effect of this treatment modality on pain perception, we would like to point to the studies that indicate that central sensitization of pain perception and defects in pain inhibition play important roles in the development and maintenance of chronic pain states (Ursin 1997, 2005, Lidbeck 2002, Eriksen & Ursin 2002, 2004, Banic et al. 2004). The treatment approaches that have demonstrated clinical effect would refer to elements like 1) lateral inhibition brought about by alternative stimuli, as touching, manual release of muscles in the painful area, move the painful area, or 2) changes in mental focus from focus on pain experience to focus on other and more pleasurable body sensations, and likewise 3) focus on coping and mastery rather than on regressive behaviour and being a passive recipient of treatment and pain killers, may be important factors.

Effect of Treatment on Level of Psychological Distress

Assessing the level of psychological distress by means of the GHQ-30 questionnaire at the time of inclusion and again at the time of one year follow-up, the main finding was that the levels of distress were reduced tin the treatment (STGT+MSCT) group, but not for the STGT group, where there was a tendency towards increased distress. Specifically, the reduction in scores for anxiety-insomnia-distress and coping tin the treatment group were highly significant, and the sub-scores for depression were reduced almost to the level of significance. The exception from this general trend, were the scores social function, where both groups experienced higher level of distress at follow-up than at inclusion. To comment on this latter result, that at first hand might seem somewhat surprising, one should bear in mind that the therapy has been limited to out patient, one-to-one encounters between the patient and the therapist, and has not included group sessions, exposure to a wider social setting or focus on social functioning in the therapy sessions. We are now starting a modified therapeutic approach, where chronic pain patients are treated in a day care program that includes a wide variety of exposures to groups and other social interaction programs.

However, the main result is the improvement with respect to anxiety, distress and coping. Although the therapy has not focused mainly on psychological symptoms such as anxiety and depressed mood states, rather on improved motor skills and reduced fear for movements. With respect to coping, the therapy has focused on dealing with the challenges related to the movements of daily living, and they have been challenged to explore the territories of new patterns of motor behaviour.

Possible Reasons for the Long-Term Positive Effect of Somatocognitive Therapy

In addition to the short term outcome of therapy after the treatment period of three months, we have demonstrated that the motor patterns and pain experience of the patients continue to improve after end of therapy, and are found to be significantly better at one year follow-up than at the immediate post-therapy assessment.

One explanation for this, that we find plausible, is that the therapy and constant practice of the cognitive and motor elements of behaviours that are so intensely rehearsed in the activities of daily living during the treatment period continue to be of use to the patient. These "toolkits" of novel approaches that the patients acquire during treatment, is now owned by the patient, who, by the success of these "tools" during active therapy, is, to a greater or lesser degree, motivated to continue the utilization of these tools is the post-treatment period. By changing the focus from pain experience towards coping of functions in activity of daily life and new motor patterns, the patient will be less fearful that movements elicit pain, conceivably by means of reduced activation of the cerebral pain neuromatrix ciruits. This implies that new strategies have been learnt, both with respect to motor skills, and with respect to the reduction of anxiety levels. When people understand *how and why* they are doing well, they can continue doing what they are doing to make themselves better. The patients will after a while in this form for treatment be their own therapists, they have learnt how to cope with respect to the challenges of daily living, and they have their own tools to use (Mensendieck 1937, Haugstad 2000, 2007).

We suggest that this pattern of further improvement of function during the follow-up period is due to a learning effect. The patients have learnt to move in a more natural and relaxed manner. The pelvic protection pattern is thus changed to a more functional and flexible use of the pelvis that promotes blood circulation and lymphatic drainage. Perhaps most importantly the pattern of respiration is changed, with an active use of the diaphragm, and thoracic and low abdominal expansion during the inspirium. The aim is that these new patterns will be automatized and integrated in the patient's new image of own body. Thus, these new motor skills are, in term, utilized without the patient conscious awareness, and they are gradually interwoven as natural parts of their new daily performance.

Somatocognitive Therapy as Contrasted to Cognitive Therapy with Chronic Pain Patients

We have, time and again, underscored the close relationship between somatocognitive therapy and cognitive psychotherapy as developed by Beck and collaborators since the 1960s. However, a word of caution is warranted: these are two approaches that are also very different. Cognitive therapy is developed as psychotherapy (Winterowd et al. 2003). As such, it only deals with the mental components of pain – the part of pain that finds itself "above the collar". It does not relate to the body, in a strict sense of the word. Even when the therapist promotes relaxation techniques, the patient only relates, in a passive way, to a restricted array of sensory input from the body. In no way is the therapist active in promoting specific use of the body, or specific strategies for experiencing alternative movement patterns, and how this leads to alternative sensations from the body. Somatocognitive therapy, again, should be understood as a hybrid of physiotherapy and psychotherapy. A wide array of sensory input from and about the body is encouraged – visual, tactile and proprioceptive among them. Even slight alterations in the postural tone or use of the extremities and shoulder and limb girdle may lead to profound alterations of, say, the respiration pattern, the free movement of abdominal and pelvic muscle groups, the position of the head in relation to the spine, the normal curvatures of the spinal column, etc. This close relation to functional anatomy is totally wanting from cognitive psychotherapy, and the theories of motor learning are also distant from the theory of cognitive therapy. On the other hand, somatocognitive therapy makes use of the proprium of cognitive therapy, in that it incorporates the understanding of dysfunctional cognitive schemata that prepares the way for negative emotional load, which again results in repressed body language. In the realm of psychiatry and therapy, somatocognitive therapy also can be said to break certain taboo areas, in that physical contact between the therapist and the patient not only is encouraged, but is seen as an absolute prerequisite in therapy.

CONCLUSION

Mensendieck physiotherapists evaluate posture, movement, gait, sitting posture and respiration with a high level of agreement when using the Standardized Mensendieck Test (SMT). The reliability is better when examining those with CPP than those with no symptoms.

The performance in all of these subtests is significantly lower in the symptomatic women's group than for the healthy controls. Thus the SMT discriminated well between patients with CPP and healthy women. These results indicate that the SMT may be useful in the evaluation of patients with CPP and other somatoform disorders.

We found a specific pattern of pain, posture, movements, muscle elasticity and reduced awareness of one's own body in women with CPP. These findings may increase our understanding of this disease.

Our study demonstrates effect of Mensendieck somatocognitive therapy on the symptom load of patients with CPP. Mensendieck somatocognitive therapy combined with standard gynecological care improved pain experience and motor functions specially the respiration and the movement of women with chronic pelvic pain better than gynecological treatment alone.

We have shown that the effect of Mensendieck somatocognitive therapy in combination with standard gynecological treatment in a group of women with CPP prevails, in that improved motor functions are lasting, and that even further progress takes place nine months after end of therapy. We suggest that this further improvement is due to a learning effect.

Suggestions for Further Research

As comments to the outcomes of this study described above, we would like to indicate that our approach might be of significance in several different areas that we have made an effort to juxtapose: Mensendieck therapy has been operationalized and developed by means of the SMT and somatocognitive therapy. This approach has been applied to the field of psychosomatic medicine in order to develop a deeper understanding of the relationship between psychological and somatic pathology, and a new approach to treating disorders like chronic pelvic pain, vulvodynia, chronic chest pain, neck and shoulder pain, low back pain and irritable bowel disease. By applying this knowledge to the field of clinical gynecology, some light may have been shed on the pathophysiology of, and treatment approach to, the chronic pelvic pain disorder. In the area of psychotherapy, application of cognitive techniques to specific somatic problems has generated new insights, and the term "somatocognitive therapy" has been coined. In terms of diagnostic classification, the possible relationships among somatoform disorders (like CPP) and disorders that involve myogenic pain (like chronic headaches) may be implicated.

In future studies we would like to clarify whether psychotherapy in addition to Mensendieck somatocognitive therapy is of importance for the treatment outcomes. This can be done by adding a third intervention group to the design, and subjecting the patients to CBT in addition to MSCT as well as STGT.

We have already initiated studies where we apply the SMT to other groups of patients (i.e., irritable bowel disorder, shoulder and neck pain), and it will be of interest if the SMT is sensitive for other patient groups.

In this study the follow up period is one year. Longer follow-up, for example five years after treatment, would clarify whether the learning effect persists.

It will also be of special interest to look at the psychometric evaluation and to the other examination to identify predictive factors with regard to degree of treatment response.

In this study, patients with major psychopathology, both with respect to symptom load (axis I) and personality traits (axis II) have been excluded. In future studies, we would like to examine whether patients displaying such symptoms respond to Mensendieck somatocognitive therapy.

Subsequent Developments and Comments

Since our study on the application of somatocognitive therapy to this particular group of gynecological patients, other authors have commented on our approach. We find the editorial comments to our last paper (Haugstad et al., 2008) in the American Journal of Obstetrics and Gynecology (AJOG) most interesting. Here it is stated that "the somatocognitive approach should be applied to patients with chronic urogenital and musculoskeletal pain", that "Gynecology departments should develop treatment programs for patients with chronic pelvic pain that incorporate a somatocognitive approach to motor analysis and therapy", and that "when no such program is available at the patient's treatment facility, she should be referred to one elsewhere". In our opinion, we may need some additional research in order to have a strong base for such wide-ranging conclusions. The research is still at its inception, and further studies, involving other centers and other target groups, should be performed. However, preliminary results from a pilot study where the current approach is applied in women with vulvodynia are promising. We have also been encouraged by several authors that have commented on and enquired into our results, that seem to find different aspects of our approach interesting, ranging from interest in the posture's effect on the tilt, position and motion of the pelvis, to the effect of a full abdominal respiration on the hemodynamics and lymphatic drainage of the pelvis minor, the concept of alexisomia and its relation to somatic dissociation, and the overall focus on showing empathy and establishing a good working alliance with the patient.

Acknowledgments

This study was made possible thanks to generous grants from Norske Kvinners Sanitetsforening and Oslo University College, with support from Oslo University Hospital Rikshospitalet and Sunnaas Hospital. We are thankful for considerable contributions over some years from Professor Ulrik Malt, Professor Per Nerdrum, Professor Harald Breivik, and Assistant Professor Elin Haakonsen, and their input is gratefully acknowledged.

References

Albert H. Psychosomatic group treatment helps women with chronic pelvic pain. *J Psychosom Obstet Gynaecol* 1999; 20:216-25.

American Psychological Association: Standards for Educational and Psycholgical Tests. Washington DC, *American Psychological Association* 1974.

Andersen P. In: Håndbok i Mensendieckgymnastikk 2.utgave, Mensendiecksystemets ledetråder i lys av nevrobiologisk kunnskap. Oslo, *Vett & Viten* 2003.

Anderson RU, Wise D, Sawyer T, Chan CA. Integration of myofacial trigger point release and paradoxical relaxation training treatment of chronic pelvic pain in men. *J Urol* 2005;174:155-60.

Anderson RU, Wise D, Sawyer T, Chan CA. Sexual dysfunction in men with chronic prostatitis/chronic pelvic pain syndrome: improvement after trigger point release and paradoxical relaxtion training. *J Urol* 2006;176:1534-8.

Anderson RU. Sexual dysfunction in men with chronic prostatitis/chronic pelvic pain syndrome: improvement after trigger point release and paradoxial relaxation training. *J Urol* 2006;176:1534-8; discussion 1538-9.

Anonymous. *The ICD-10 classification of mental and behavioural disorders. Clinical descriptions and diagnostic guidelines of women with chronic pelvic pain.* Geneva, World Health Organization, 1992;160-169.

Anonymous. IASP task force on taxonomy. *Classification of chronic pain.* Seattle, IASP Press 1994; pp 209-214.

Apkarian AV, Bushnell MC, Treede RD, Zubieta JK. Human brain mechanisms of pain perception and regulation and disease. *E J Pain* 2005;9: 463-484.

Baker PK. Musculoskeletal origins of chronic pelvic pain. Diagnosis and Treatment. *Obstetrics Gynecol Clin N Am* 1993;20:719-43.

Bakke A, Malt UF. Social function and general well-being in patients treated with clean intermittent catheterization *J Psychosom Res* 1993; 37: 371-380

Banic B, Petersen-Felix S, Andersen OK, Radanov BP, Villiger PM, Arendt-Nielsen L, Curatolo M. Evidence for spinal cord hypersensitivity in chronic pain after whiplash injury and in fibromyalgia. *Pain* 2004;107:7-15.

Baranowski AP. Chronic pelvic pain. *Best Pract Res Clin Gastroenterol* 2009;23:593-610.

Bates SM, Hill VA, Anderson JB, Chapple CR, Spence R, Ryan C, Talbot MD. A prospective, randomized, double-blind trial to evaluate the role of a short reducing course of oral corticosteroid therapy in the treatment of chronic prostatitis/chronic pelvic pain syndrome. *BJU International* 2007; 99: 355-9.

Beard RW, Reignald PW, Wadsworth J. Clinical features of women with chronic lower abdominal pain and pelvic congestion. *Br J Obstet Gynaecol* 1988;95:153-61.

Beck AT. *Cognitive therapy and the emotional disorders.* New York, International Universities Press 1976.

Benestad HB, Laake P. *Forskningsmetode i medisin og biofag.* Oslo, Gyldendal 2004.

Berberich HJ, Ludwig M. Psychosomatic aspects of the chronic pelvic pain syndrome. *Urologe* A 2004;43:254-60.

Bergman J, Zeitlin SI. Prostatitis and chronic prostatitis/chronic pelvic pain syndrome. *Expert Rev Neurother*. 2007 Mar;7(3):301-7.

Birmauer N, Flor H, Cevey B, Dworkin B, Miller NE. Behavioural treatment and scoliosis and kyphosis. *J Psychosom Res* 1994;38:623-8.

Bodden-Heidrich R, Kuppers V, Beckmann MW, Rechenberger I, Bender HG. Chronic pelvic pain syndrome (CPPS) and chronic vulvar pain syndrome

(CVPS): evaluation of psychosomatic aspects. *Psychosom Med Psychother* 1999;45:372-389.

Bodden-Heidrich R, Kuppers V, Beckmann MW, Rechenberger I, Bender HG. *Chronic pelvic pain and chronic vulvodynia as multifactorial psychosomatic disease syndromes: results of a psychometric and clinical study taking into account musculoskeletal diseases.* Zentralbl Gynakol 1999;121:389-9.

Bodden-Heidrich R. *Chronic pelvic pain syndrome- a multifactioral syndrome.* Zentralbl Gynakol 2001;23:10-7.

Bodden-Heidrich R, Hilberink M, Frommer J. *Psychosomatic aspects of urogynaecology: model considerations on the pathogenesis, diagnosis and therapy.* Zentral Gynakol 2004;126:237-43.

Borg-Stein J. Treatment of fibromyalgia, myofascial pain, and related disorders *Phys Med Rehabil Clin N Am* 2006;17:491-510

Breen J. Transitions in the Concept of Chronic Pain. *Nurs Sci* 2002;24:48-59.

Bunkan BH. *Muskelspenninger og kroppsbilde. Undersøkelse og behandling.* Oslo, Universitetsforlaget AS 1985.

Bunkan BH, Moen O, Opjordsmoen S, Moen O, Friis S. What are the basic dimensions of respiration? A psychometric evaluation of The Comprehensive Body Examination II. *Nord J Psychiatry* 1999;53:361-369.

Bunkan BH. *The Comprehensive Body Examination.* Manual. Oslo, Norwegian University Press 2000.

Bunkan BH, Ljunggren AE, Opjordsmoen S, Moen O, Friis S. What are the basic dimensions of movements? A psychometric evaluation of the Comprehensive Body Examination III. *North J Pschiatry* 2001;55:33-40.

Bunkan BH, Moen O, Opjordsmoen S, Ljunggren AE, Friis S. Interrater reliability of the comprehensive body examination. *Physiotherapy Theory and Practice* 2002;18:121-129.

Bunkan BH. *The resource-oriented body examination.* A manual, Oslo Gyldendal 2003.

van Bussel JC, Spitz B, Demyttenaere K. Women's mental health before, during, and after pregnancy: a population-based controlled study. *Birth* 2006; 33: 297-302.

Butler AC, Beck JS. Cognitive Therapy Outcomes: A Review of Meta-Analyses. *Tidsskrift for Norsk Psykologforening* 2001;38:698-706.

Byrne P. Psychiatric morbidity in a gynaecology clinic: an epidemiological survey. *Br J Psychiatry* 1984;144:28-34.

Campbell A, Walker J, Farrell G. Confirmatory factor analysis of the GHQ-12: can I see that again? *Austr NZ J Psychiatry* 2003;37:475-83.

Campbell LC, Clauw DJ, Keefe FJ. Persistent pain and depression: a biopsychosocial perspective. *Biol Psychiatry* 2003;54:399-409.

Carr JH, Sheperd RB. *Neurological rehabilitation – Optimizing motor performance*. Oxford, Butterworth –Heineman 2010.

Chang L. Brain responses to visceral and somatic stimuli in irritable bowel syndrome: a central nervous system disorder. *Gastroenterol Clin North Am* 2005;34:271-9.

Chaaya MM, Bogner HR, Gallo JJ, Leaf PJ. The association of gynecological symptoms with psychological distress in women of reproductive age: a survey from gynecology clinics in Beirut, Libanon. *J Psychosom Obstet Gynaecol* 2003;24:175-84.

Ching HL, Burke V, Stuckey BG. Quality of life and psychological morbidity in women with polycystic ovary syndrome: body mass index, age and the provision of patient information are significant modifiers. *Clin Endocrinol* 2007;66:373-9.

Cornel EB, van Haast EP, Schaarsberg RW, Greels J. The effect of bio-feedback physiotherapy in men with Chronic Pelvic Pain Syndrome Type III. *Eur Urol* 2005;47:607-11.

Crooks LK. Assessing Pain and the Joint Commission Pain Standards. *Top Emerg Med* 2002;2:1-9.

Diatchenko L, Nackley AG, Slade GD, Fillingim RB, Maixner W. Idiopatic pain disorders – pathways of vulnerability. *Pain* 2006;123:226-30.

Dick ML. Chronic pelvic pain in women: assessment and management. *Aust Fam Physician* 2004;33:971-6

Dimitrakov JD, Kaplan SA, Kroenke K, Jackson JL, Freeman MR. Management of chronic prostatitis/chronic pelvic pain syndrome: an evidence-based approach. *Urology* 2006;67:881-8.

Duffy S. Chronic pelvic pain: defining the scope of the problem. *Int J Gyn Obst* 2001;74:3-7.

Ehlert U, Heim C, Hellhammer DH. *Chronic Pelvic Pain as a Somatoform Disorder Psychother Psychosom* 1999;68:87-94.

Ekerholt K, Bergland A. The first encounter with Norwegian psychomotor physiotherapy: patient's experiences, a basis for knowledge. *Scand J Public Health* 2004;32:403-10.

Engman M, Lindehammar H, Wijma B. Surface electromyography diagnostics in women with partial vaginismus with or without vulvar vestibulitis and in asymptomatic women. *J Psychosom Obstet Gynaecol* 2004;25:281-94.

Erikson E, Nordwall RPT, Kurlberg G. Effects on Body Awareness Therapy in Patients with Irritable Bowel syndrome. *Adv Phys* 2002;4:125-135.

Eriksen HR, Ursin H. Senzitization and subjective health complaints. *Scand J Psychol* 2002;43:189-96.

Eriksen HR, Ursin H. Subjective health complaints, sensitization, and sustained cognitive activation. *J Psychosom Res* 2004;56:445-8

Facchini S, Muellbacher W, Battaglia F, Boroojerdi B, Halett M. Focal enhancement of motor cortex excitability during motor imagery: a transcranial magnetic stimulation study. *Acta neurol scand* 2002;105:146-51.

Fitts PM, Posner MI. *Human performance.* Belmont, CA: Brooks/Cole Publishing Company 1967.

Fitts PM. The Information Capacity of the Human Motor System in Controlling the Amplitude of Movement. Journal of Experimental Psychology: 1954; 47:381-391. *Reprint Journal of Experimental Psychology: General,* 1992;121:262-269.

FitzGerald MP, Kotarinos R. Rehabilitation of the short pelvic floor. I: Background and patient evaluation. *Int Urogyn J Pelvic Floor Dysfunct* 2003;14:261-8.

Fitzgerald MP. Can chronic pelvic pain in men be treated with myofacial trigger point release and paradoxiacal relaxation training? *J Urol* 2005;174:155-160.

Flanagan JR, Vetter P; Johansson RS; Wolpert DM. Prediction precedes control in motor learning. *Curr Biol.* 2003;13:146-50.

Freeman A, Greenwood V. *Cognitive therapy. Applications in Psychiatric and Medical settings.* New York, Human sciences press 1987.

Friis S, Skatteboe UB, Hope MK, Vaglum P. Body Awareness Group Therapy for Patients with Personality Disorders. 2. Evaluation of the Body Awareness Rating Scale. *Psychother Psychosom* 1989;51,18-24.

Friis S, Bunkan BH, Ljunggren AE, Moen O, Opjordsmoen S. What are the basic of dimensions of body posture? An empirical evaluation of the Comprehensive Body Examination. I. *Nord J Psychiatry* 1998;52:319-326.

Friis S, Bunkan BH, Opjordsmoen S, Moen O, Ljunggren AE. The Comprehensive Body Examination (CBE): From global impressions to specific sub-scales. *Advances in Physiotherapy* 2002;4:161-168.

Gallagher RM. Rational polypharmacy in integrated pain treatment. Am *J Phys Med Rehabil* 2005;84:64-76.

Gallagher RM, Verma S. Biopsychosocial pain medicine: Integrating medical, psychiatric and behavioural therapies. *Semin Neurosurg* 2004;15:31-46.

Gard G. Body awareness therapy for patients with fibromyalgia and chronic pain. *Disability and Rehabilitation* 2005;27:725-728.

Gentile AM. A working model of skill acquistion to teaching. *Quest* 1972;17:3-23.

Gentile AM. Implicit and explicit processes during acquisition of functional skills. *Scand J Occup Therapy* 1998;5:7-16.

Giubilei G, Mondaini N, Minervini A, Saieva C, Lapini A, Serni S, Batroletti R, Carini M. Psysical activity of men with chronic prostatitis/chronic pelvic pain syndrome not satisfied with conventional treatments –could it represent a valid option? The physical activity and male pelvic pain trial: a double-blind, randomized study. *J Urol* 2007;177:159-65.

Goldapple K, Segal Z, Garson C, Lau M, Bieling P, Kennedy S, Mayberg H. *Modulation of cortical-limbic pathways in major depression: treatment-specific effects of cognitive behaviour therapy.*

Goldberg D, Williams P. *A user's guide to the General Health Questionnaire.* Windsor NFER-Nelson 1988.

Goldby LJ, Moore AP, Doust J, Trew ME. A randomized controlled trial investigating the efficiency of musculoskeletal physiotherapy on chronic low back disorder. *Spine* 2006;31:1083-93.

Grace VM, Zondervan KT. Pelvic pain in New Zealand: prevalence, pain severity, diagnosis and use of the health services. Australian and *New Zealand Journal of Public Health* 2004;28:369-75.

Grace VM. Problems of communication, diagnosis and treatment experienced by women using the New Zealand health services for chronic pelvic pain. *A quantitative analysis. Health Care Women Int.* 1995:66;117-127.

Green C, Tait R, Gallagher RM. The unequal burden of pain: disparities and differences. *Pain Med* 2004;6:1-2.

Greco CD. Management of adolecent chronic pelvic pain from endometriosis: a pain center perspective. *J Ped Adol Gyn* 2003;16:17-19.

Gullacksen AC, Lidbeck J. The life adjustment process in chronic pain: Psychosocial assessment and clinical implications. *Pain Res Manage* 2004;9:145-153.

Gunter J. Chronic Pelvic Pain: An Integrated Approach to Diagnosis and Treatment. *Obstetrical and Gynecological Survey* 2003;58:615-23.

Gyllensten AL, Ekdahl C, Hansson L. Validity of the Body Awareness scale-helath (BAS-H). *Scand J Caring Sci* 1999; 13: 217-26.

Gyllensten AL, Gard G, Salford E, Ekdahl C. Interaction between patient and physiotherapist: a qualitative study reflecting the physiotherapist's perspective. *Physiother Res Int.* 1999;4:89-109.

Gyllensten AL, Ovesson MN, Lindstrom I, Hansson L, Ekdahl C. Reliability of Body Awareness Scale-Health. *Scand J Caring Sci.* 2004;18:213-9.

Halvorsen G. Mensendiecks historie. *Vett & Viten* 2009.

Hamaoui A, Do M, Pupard L, Bouisset S. Does respiration perturb body balance more in chronic low back pain subjects than in healthy subject? *Clin Biomech* 2002;17:548-50.

Haugstad GK. Behandling av psykosomatiske lidelser. *Fysioterapeuten* 1999;66:13-17.

Haugstad GK. Utvikling og validering av en standardisert, kvantifisert Mensendieck test. Anvendelse av testen ved fysioterapiundersøkelse av kroniske smertepasienter. *Hovedfagsoppgave Det medisinske fakultet Universitetet i Oslo*; 2000.

Haugstad GK; Haugstad TS; Leganger S, Kirste UM; Malt UF. A controlled, randomized intervention study of patients with chronic low abdominal pain. *J Psychosom Res* 2000;48:235.

Haugstad GK, Malt UF, Leganger S, Kirse UM, Haugstad TS. *Mensendieck somatocognitive therapy*. Platform presentation at the 25th World Conference in Psychotherapy. Trondheim, August 2002.

Haugstad GK, Haugstad TS, Kirste UM, Leganger S, Wojniusz S, Klemmetsen I, Malt UF. Posture, movement patterns, and body awareness in women with chronic pelvic pain. *Journal of Psychosomatic Research* 2006b;61:637-644.

Haugstad GK, Haugstad TS, Kirste UM, Leganger S, Hammel B, Klemmetsen I, Malt UF. Reliability and validity of a standardized Mensendieck physiotherapytest (SMT). *Physiotherapy Theory and Practice* 2006a; 22:189-205.

Haugstad GK, Haugstad TS, Kirste UM, Leganger S, Hammel B, Klemmetsen I, Malt UF. Mensendieck somatocognitive therapy as treatment approach to chronic pelvic pain. Results of a randomized controlled intervention study. *Am J Obst & Gyn* 2006c;196:1303-10

Haugstad GK. "Mensendieck Somtocognitive therapy of women with gynaecological unexplained chronic pelvic pain. " *Doctoral Thesis Faculty of Oslo* 2007

Haugstad GK, Haugstad TS, Kirste UM, Leganger S, Wojniusz S, Klemetsen I, Malt UF. Continuing improvement of chronic pelvic pain in women after short-term Mensendieck somatocognitive therapy: results of 1-year follow-up study. *Am J Obst & Gyn;*199:615.e1-615.e8.

Havermark AM, Languis-Eklof A. Long-term follow up of a physical therapy programme for patients with fibromyalgia syndrome. *Scand J Caring Sci.* 2006 Sep;20:315-22.

Hersoug AG. Quality of working alliance in psychotherapy: Therapist contribution. *Psychologist Psychoanalyst* 2002;22:18-20.

Hetrick DC, Ciol MA Rothman I, Turner JA, Frest M, Berger RE. Muscloskeletal dysfunction in men with chronic pelvic pain syndrome type III: A case-control study. *J Urolology* 2003;170:828-831.

Higgins S. Motor skill acquisition. *Physical Therapy* 1991;71:123-139.

Hilden M, Schei B, Swahnberg K, Halmesmäki E, Langhoff-Roos J, Offerdal K, Pikarinen U, Sidenius K, Steingrimsdottir T, Stoum-Hinsverk H, Wijma B. A history of sexual abuse and health: a Nordic multicentre study. *BJOG* 2004; 111: 1121-7.

Hodges NJ, Franks IM. Modelling coaching practice: the role of instruction and demonstration. *Journal of Sports Sciences* 2002;20:793-811.

Hofbauer RK, Rainville P, Duncan GH, Bushnell MC. Cortical representation of the sensory dimension of pain. *J Neurophysiol* 2001;86:402-11.

Hoffart A, Nordahl HM. Kvalitetssikring av kognitiv terapi: En modell for veiledning. *Tidsskrift for Norsk Psykologforening* 2001;8:707-717.

Howard FM. Chronic pelvic pain. *Obstet Gynecol* 2003;101:594-611.

Horwitz-Stern R, Smolin Y. Chronic pelvic pain. Chapter 35. In: Blumenfield M, Strain JJ. *Psychosomatic Medicine*. Philadelphia USA, Lippincott Williams & Wilkins 2006.

Huppert FA, Walters DA; Day NE, ElliottJB: The factor structure of the General Health Questionnaire (GHQ-30*). Br J Psychiatry* 1989;155:178-185.

Jain S, Janssen K, DeCelle S. Alexander technique and Feldenkrais method: a critical overview. *Phys Med Rehab Clin N Am* 2004;15:811-25.

Jamieson DJ, Steege JF. The prevalence of dysmenorrhoea, dyspareunia, pelvic pain and irritable bowel syndrome in primary care practices. *Obstet Gynecol* 1996;87:332-7.

Jarell, J. Myofacial dysfunction in the pelvis. *Curr Pain Headache Rep* 2004;8:452-6.

Jensen MP, Karoly P, Braver S. The measurement of clinical pain intensity: a comparison of six methods. *Pain* 1986;27:117-126.

Kames LD, Rapkin AJ, Naliboff BD. Effectiveness of an interdisiplinary pain management program for the treatment of chronic pelvic pain. *Pain* 1990;41:41-46.

Kanbara K, Mitani Y, Fukunaga M, Ishino S, Takebayashi N, Nakai Y. Paradoxial results of psychophysiological stress profile in functional somatic syndrome: correaltion between subjective tension score and objective stress response. *Appl Psychophysiol Biofeedback* 2004;29:255-68.

Kelly S, Lloyd D, Nurmikko T, Roberts N. Retrieving Autobiographical Memories of Painful Events Activates Cingulate Cortex and Inferior Frontal Gyrus. *J Pain* 2007;8:307-14.

Kendall SA, Brolin-Magnusson K, Søren B, Gerdle B, Henriksson KG. A Pilot Study of Body Awareness Programs in the Treatment of Fibromyalgia Syndrome. *Arthritis Care and Research* 2000;13:304-307.

Kirste UM, Haugstad GK, Leganger S, Blomhoff S, Malt UF. *Chronic pelvic pain in women*. Tidsskrift Nor Læegeforen. 2002;122:1223-7.

Klemmetsen I. *The Mensendieck System of Functional Movements*. Oslo, Vett & Viten AS 2005.

Kotarinos RK. Pelvic floor physical therapy in urogynecologic disordres. *Curr Women Health Rep* 2003;3:334-9.

Kulkarni B, Bentley DE, Elliott R, Youell P, Watson A, Derbyshire SW, Frackowiak KJ, Jones AK. Attention to pain lokalization and unpleasantness discriminates the functions of the medial and lateral pain systems. *Eur J Neurosci* 2005;21:3133-42.

Kvåle A, Ljunggren AE, Johnsen TB. Examination of movement in patients with longlasting musculoskeletal pain: reliability and validity. *Physiotherapy Research International* 2003a;8:36-52.

Kvåle A, Johnsen TB, Ljunggen AE. Examination of respiration in Patients with longlasting musculoskeletal pain: Reliability and Validity. *Adv Phys* 2002;4:169-81.

Kvåle A, Skouen JS, Ljunggren AE. Discrimintive validity of Global Physiotherapy Examination (GPE-52) in patients with longlasting musculoskeletal pain verus healthy persons. *J Musculoskel Pain* 2003b;11.

Kvåle A. *Measurement properties of a Global Physiotherapy Examination in patients with long-lasting musculoskeletal pain*. Doctoral thesis. Section of Physiotherapy Science Department of Public Health and Primary Health Care. Faculty of Medicine University of Bergen, 2003c.

Kvåle A, Skouen JS, Ljunggren AE. Sensitivity to change and responssiveness of the global physiotherapy examination (GPE-52) in patients with long-lasting musculoskeletal pain. *Phys Ther* 2005;85:712-26.

Lambert MJ, Bergin AE, Garfield SL. Introduction and historical overview. In MJ Lambert (Ed.), Bergin and Garfield's Handbook of Psychotherapy and Behavior Change. New York: Wiley; 2004

Lamoth CJC, Daffertshofer A, Meijer O, Moseley GL, Wuisman PIJM, Beek PJ. Effects of experimentally induced pain and fear of pain on trunk coordination and back muscle activity during walking. *Clinical Biomechanics* 2004;19:551-563.

Learman LA, Kuppermann M, Gates E, Gregorich SE, Lewis J, Washington AE. Predictors of hysterectomy in women with common pelvic problems: a uterine survival analysis.*J Am Coll Surg* 2007; 204:633-41

Lidbeck J. Group therapy for somatization disorders in general practice: Effectiveness of a short cognitive- behavioural treatment mode. *Acta Psychiatrica Scandinavica* 1997;96:14-24.

Lidbeck J. Central hyperexcitability in chronic musculoskeletal pain: a conceptual breakthrough with multiple clinical implications. *Pain Res Manag* 2002;7(2):81-92.

Lingsten K, Halvorsen G. *Sykegrep; behandlingsgrep innenfor Mense-ndiecktradisjonen.* Oslo, Vett & Viten AS 2001

Linton SJ, Nordin E. A 5-year follow-up evaluation of health and economic consequences of an early cognitive behavioral intervention for back pain: a randomized, controlled trial. *Spine* 2006;31:853-8.

Loeser JD, Turk DC. Multidisciplinary pain management. In: Loeser JD, Butler SH, Chapman RC, Turk DC eds. *Bonica's Management of Pain.* 3rd ed. Philadelphia , PA: Lippincott Williams 6 Wilkins; 2001:2069-2079.

Maigne JY, Chatellier G, Faou ML, Archambeau M. The treatment of chronic coccydynia with intrarectal manipulation: a randomized controlled study. *Spine* 2006;15:621-7.

Malt UF. The validity of the General Health Questionnaire in a sample of accidentally injured adults. *Acta Psychiatr Scand* 1989; 80 (Suppl. 355): 103-112.

Malt UF, Nerdrum P, Oppedal B, Gundersen R, Holte M, Løne J. Physical and mental problems attributed to dental amalgam fillings. A descriptive study of 99 self-referred patients compared with 272 controls. *Psychosom Med* 1997;59:32-41

Malmgren-Olsson EB, Branhold IB. A comparison between three physiotherapy approaches with regard to health-related factors in patients with non-specific musculoskeletal disorders. *Disabil Rehabil* 2002; 24:308-17.

Mathias SD, Kuppermann M, Liberman RF, Steege JF: Chronic pelvic pain, prevalence, health-related quality of life, and economic correlates. *Obstet Gynecol* 1996;87:332-7.

Mattson M, Wikman M, Dahlgren L, Mattson B. Physiotherapy as Empowerment-Treating Women with Chronic Pelvic Pain. *Advances in Physiotherapy* 2000;2:125-143.

Mayou RA. Somatization. *Psychother Psychosom* 1993:59;69-83.

Mayou RA, Bryant B, Sanders D, Bass C, Klimes I, Forfar C. A controlled trial of cognitive behavioural therapy for non-cardiac chest pain. *Psychol Med* 27;1021-31.

McCaffery M. Nursing *Practice theories Related to Cognition, Bodily Pain, and Man-Environment Interaction.* Los Angeles, Calif UCLA Student Store;1968.

McCaffery M, Pasero C. Practical nondrug approaches to pain. In: McCaffery M, Pasero C eds. *Pain: Clinical Manual*, 2nd ed. St. Louis: Mosby; 1999:399-427.

Mensendieck BM. Bewegungsprobleme. *Die Gestaltung schøner Arme.* München, F. Bruckman 1927.

Mensendieck BM. *The Mensendieck system of functional exercises,* volume I. Portland, Maine;1937:The Southworth - Anthoensen Press

Mensendieck BM. *Look better, feel better.* New York, Harper & Brothers 1954.

Merskey H, Bogduk N. *Classification of Chronic Pain. Descriptions of Chronic Pain Syndromes and Definitions of Pain Terms*, 2nd edn. Seattle, IASP Press 1994.

Meyer-Lidenberg A. Impact of prosocial neutopeptides on human brain function. *Prog Brain Res* 2008;170:463-70

Montenegro ML, Mateues-Vasconcelos EC, Rosa E Silva JC, Dos Reis FJ, Nogueira AA, Poli-Neto OB. Postural changes in women with chronic pelvic pain: a case control study. *BMC Musculoskelet Disord* 2009; 7:10:82

Mosely GL. A pain neuromatrix approach to patients with chronic pain. *Man Ther* 2003;8:130-140.

Nadler RB. Bladder training biofeedback and pelvic floor myalgia. *Urology* 2002;60:42-44.

Nerdrum P. Training of emphatic communication for helping professionals. *Doctoral dissertation.* Oslo University 2000.

Nerdrum P, Rønnestad MH. The trainees'perspective. A qualitive study of learning emphatic communication in Norway. *The Counseling Psychologist* 2002;30:609-629.

Nerdrum P, Rønnestad MH. Changes in Therapists' Conceptualization and Practice of Therapy Following empathy Training. *The Clinical Supervisor* 2003;20:37-61.

Nicholson A, Fuhrer R, Marmot M. Psychological distress as a predictor of CHD events in men: the effect of persistence and components of risk. *Psychosom Med* 2005;67:522-30.

Nijenhuis ERS. *Somatoform dissociation: phenomena, measurement and theoretical issues*. New York: WWNorton & Company; 2004.

Osborne TL, Raichle KA, Jensen MP. Psychologic interventions for chronic pain. *Phys Med Rehabil Clin N Am*. 2006;17:415-33.

Ohayon MM, Schatzberg AF. Using chronic pain to predict depressive morbidity in the general population. *Arch Gen Psychiatry* 2003;60:39-47.

Peters AAW, Dorst E van, Jelli B, Zuuren E van, Hermans J, Trimbos JB. A randomized clinical trial to compare two different approaches in women with chronic pelvic pain. *Obstetrics and Gynecology* 1992; 7:740-44.

Phillips ML, Gregory LJ, Cullen S, Cohen S, Ng V, Andrew C. The effect of negative emotional context on neural and behavioural reponses to oesophageal stimulation. *Brain* 2003;126:669-84.

Pyszel A, Malyszczak K, Pyszel K, Andrzejak R, Szuba A. Disability, psychological distress and quality of life in breast cancer survivors with arm lymphedema. *Lymphology* 2006;39:185-92.

Rakin G, Stokes M. Reliability of assessment tools in rehabilitation: an illustration of appropriate stastistical analyes. *Clin Rehabil* 1998;12:187-199

Rapkin AJ, Kames LD. The pain management approach to chronic pelvic pain. *J Reprod Med* 1987;32:323-7.

Reich W. The Function of the orgasm. London, Panther Books 1961.

Reinecke AM, Dattilio FM, Freeman A. *Cognitive therapy with children and adolecents*. New York; The Guilford Press 1996.

Rempel DM, Krause M, Goldberg R, Benner D, Hudes M, Goldner GU. A randomised controlled trial evaluating the effects of two workstations intervention on upper body pain and incident musculoskelatal disorders among computer operators. *Occup Environ Med* 2006;63:300-6.

Rigault NB. *Mensendieck-systemet i et didatisk perspektiv - på jakt etter røtter*. Hovedfagsoppgave. Universitetet i Oslo, 1989.

Rosenbaum TY, Owens A. The role of pelvic floor physical therapy in the treatment of pelvic and genital pain related sexual dysfunction. *J Sex Med* 2008; 5:513-523.

Rosmalen JGM, Neeleman J, Bans ROB, de Jonge P. The association between neuroticism and self-reported common somatic symptoms in a population cohort. *J Psychosom Res* 2007;62:305-11.

Roxendal G. Psychosomatically oriented physiotherapy. In: Sivik T & Theorell T, editor, *Psychosomtic medicine*. Lund: Studentlitteratur; 1995.

Ryum T, Stile T.C. Betydningen av den terapeutiske allianse: en studie av alliansen prediktive validitet. *Tidsskrift for Norsk Psykologforening* 42;998-1003.

Salvesen KA, Morkved S. Randomised controlled trial of pelvic floor muscle training during pregnancy. *BMJ* 2004:329:378-380.

Schachter S, Singer J. Cognitive, social and physiological determinants of emotional state. *Psychol Review* 1962;69:379-99.

Schaeffer AJ. Etiology and management of chronic pelvic pain syndrome in men. *Urology* 2004;63:75-83.

Schlinger M. Feldenkrais Method, Alexander Technique, and yoga-body awareness therapy in performing arts. *Phys Med Rehab Clin N AM* 2006; 17.865-75.

Schonstein E, Kenny DT, Keating J, Koes B, Herbert RD. Physical conditioning, work hardening and functional restoration for workers with back and neck pain: a cochrane systematic review. *Spine* 2003a;28:391-5.

Schonstein E, Kenny DT, Keating J, Koes BW. Work condition, work hardening and functional restoation for workers with back and neck pain. *Cochrane Database Syst Rev*. 2003b;1:CD001822.(b)

Schontz FC. Fundamentals of Research In *The Behavioral Sciences. Principles and Practice.* 1986; American Psychatric Press, Inc.

Sharp DJ. Validation of the 30-item General Health Questionnaire in early pregnancy. *Psychol Med* 1988;18:503-7.

Sharpe M. Cognitive behavioural therapies in the treatment of functional somatic symptoms. *Treatment of functional somatic symptoms*. 1995;7.122-143. Oxford:Oxford University Press.

Shields SA, Mallory ME, Simon A. The Body Awareness Questionnaire: Reliability and validity. *J Pers Assess* 1989; 53: 802-15.

Shrout PE, Fleiss JL. Intraclass correlations uses in assessing rater reliability. *Psychological Bulletin* 1979;86:420-428.

Sidentopf F, Kentenich H. *Chronic pelvic pain in women*. Zentral Gynakol 2004;126:61-6.

Silverstein B. Gender differences in the prevalence of clinical depression: the role played by depression associated with somatic symptoms. *Am J Psychiatry* 1999;156:480-2.

Silverstein B. Gender differences in the prevalence of somatic versus pure depression: a replication. *Am J Psychiatry* 2002;159:1051-2.

Skatteboe U. Basal kroppskjennskap og bevegelsesharmoni. Videreutvikkling av undersøkelsesmetoden *Body Awareness Rating Scale,* BARS-Bevegelsesharmoni. Oslo; Høgskolen i Oslo, HiO publikasjon, 2000.

Skouen JS, Grasdal AL, Haldorsen EMH, Ursin H. Relative cost-effectiveness of extensive and light multidisciplinary programs for chronic low back pain patients on long- term sick leave. A randomized controlled study. *Spine* 2002;27:901-909.

Slocumb JC. Neurological factors in chronic pelvic pain: Trigger points in the abdominal pelvic pain syndrom. *Am J Obst Gynecol* 1987;149:536-543.

Smeets RJ, Vlaeyen JW, Kester AD, Knottnerus JA. Reduction of pain catastrophing mediates the outcome of both physical and cognitive-behavioral treatment in chronic low back pain. *J Pain* 2006;7:261-71.

Souter VL, Hopton JL, Penney GC, Templeton AA. Survey of psychological health in women with infertility. *J Psychosom Obestet Gynaecol* 2002;23:41-9.

Staud R, Domingo M. Evidence for abnormal pain processing in fibromyalgia syndrome. *Pain Med.* 2001;2:208-15.

Staud R, Vierck CJ, Robinson ME, Price DV. *Effects of the N-methyl-D-aspartate receptor anatagonist dextromethorphan on temporal summation of pain are similar in fibromyalgia patients and normal control subjects.* 2005;6:323-32.

Stegner AJ, Tobar DA, Kane MT. Generalizability of change scores on the Body Awareness Scale. *Measure phys edu exercise science* 1999;3:125-40.

Sterling M, Jull G, Vicenzino B, Kenardy J, Darnell R. Physical and psychological factors predict outcome following whiplash injury. *Pain* 2005; 114: 141-8.

Stones RW, Mountfield J. Management of chronic pelvic pain in women. *Cochrane Database Syst Rev* 1998;2:1.

Stuge B, Veierod MB, Laerum E, Vollestad N. The effecacy of treatment program focusing on specific stabilizing exercises for pelvic girdle pain after pregnancy: a two- year follow-up of a randomized clinical trial. *Spine* 2004;15:197-203.

Soukup MG, Glomsrød B, Lønn JH, Bø K, Larsen S. The Effect of Mensendieck Exercise Program as Secondary Prophylaxis for Recurrent Low Back Pain. A randomized, Controlled Trial With 12-Month Follow-up. *Spine* 1999;24:1585-1591.

Sundsvold MØ, Vaglum P, Denstad K. *Global fysioterapeutisk muskel-undersøkelse.* Oslo, Private publishing company 1982.

Sundsvold MØ, Vaglum P, Denstad K. Muscular pain and psychopathology: evaluation by the GMP method. International Perspectives in Physical Therapy. In: Michel Th (Red.) *Volume on Pain.* London, Churchill Livingstone; 1985:18-47.

Tu FF, As-Sanie S, Steege JF. Musculoskeletal causes of chronic pelvic pain: a systematic review of diagnosis: Part I. *Obstet Gynecol Surv* 2005;60:379-85.

Tu FF, As- Sanie S, Steege JF. Musculoskeletal causes of chronic pelvic pain: a systematic review of existing therapies: part II. *Obstet Gynecol Surv.* 2005;60:474-83.

Tu FF, As-Sanie S, Steege JF. Prevalence of musculoskeletal disorders in female chronic pelvic pain clinic. *J Reprod Med* 2006;51:185-9.

Tu FF, Holt J, Gonzales J, Fitzgerald CM. Physical therapy evaluations of patients with chronic pelvic pain: a controlled study. *Am J Obstet Gynecol* 2008;198:272e1-7.

Turk DC, Okifuji A, Sherman J. Behavioral aspects of low back pain. In: Taylor JR, Twomey L. *Physical Therapy of the Low Back. 3rd ed.* New York, NY: Churchill Livingstone, 2000:351-383.

Turk DC. Cognitive-behavioral approach to the treatment of chronic pain patients. *Reg Anesth Pain med* 2003;28:573-9.

Ursin H. Senzitization, somatization and subjective health complaints. A review. *Int J Behav Med* 1997;4:105-116.

Ursin H, Eriksen HR. Sensitization, subjective health complaints, and sustained arousal. *Ann N Y Acad Sci* 2001;933:119-29.

Ursin H. Press stop to start: the role of inhibition for choice and health. *Psychoneuroendocrinology* 2005;30:1059-65.

Villemure C, Bushnell MC. Cognitive modulation of pain: how do attention and emotion influence pain processing? *Pain* 2002;95:195-9.

Vlayen JWS, Crombez G, Goubert L. Science and psychology of pain. In; Breivik H, Schipley M, editors. *Pain best practice and research compendium*. London: Elsevier: 2007.p.7-15.

Warnock JK, Clayton AH. Chronic episodic disorders in women. *Psychiatr Clin North Am* 2003;26:725-740.

Weiner D, Peterson B, Keefe F. Chronic pain-associated behaviors in the nursing home: resident versus caregiver perceptions. *Pain* 1999;80:577-88.

Wejenborg PP, Ter Kuile MM, Stones W. A cognitive based assessment of women with chronic pelvic pain. J Psychosom Obst Gyn 2009;30:262-8.

Wennemer U, Borg-Stein J, Gomba L, Delaney B, Rothmund A, Barlow D, Breeze G, Thompson A. Functionally oriented rehabilitation program for patients with fibromyalgia: preliminary results. *Am J Phys Med Rehabil.* 2006;85:659-66.

Wesselmann U, Czakanski PP. Pelvic Pain: A Chronic Visceral Pain Syndrome. *Current Pain and Headache Reports* 2001;5:13-19.

Wigers SH, Finset. A. Rehabilitation of chronic myofascial pain disorders. *Tidsskr Nor Laegeforen.* 2007;127:604-8.

Wijma B, Schei B, Swahnberg K, Hilden M, Offerdal K, Pikarinen U, Sidenious K, Steingrimsdottir T, Stoum H, Halmesmäki E. Emotional, physcial, and sexual abuse in patients visiting gynaecology clinics: a Nordic cross-sectional study. *Lancet* 2003;361:2107-13.

Winkelstein BA. Mechanisms of central sensitization, neuroimmunology & injury biomechanisms in persistent pain: implications for musculoskeletal disorders. *J eletromyogr Kinesiol* 2004;14:87-93.

Winterowd C, Beck AT, Gruener D. *Cognitve Therapy with Chronic Pain Patients.* New York Springer Publishing Company 2003.

Wojniusz S. Association between personality traits and bodily findings. An explorative pilot study. *Master thesis Institute of Nursing and Health Sciences Faculty of medicine* University of Oslo 2006.

Worsley A, Walters WA, Wood EC. Responses of Australian patients with gynaecological disorders to the General Health Questionnaire: a factor analytic study. *Psychol Med.* 1978;8:131-8.

Yutzy SH. Somatization. In: Blumenfield M, Strain JJ. *Psychosomatic Medicine.* Philadelphia, Lippincott Williams &Wilkins 2006;537-543.

Zondervan KT. The community prevalence of chronic pelvic pain in women and associated illness behaviour. *Br J Gen Pract* 2001;51:541-547.

Zondervan, KT, Yudkin PL, Vessey MP, Dawes MG, Balow DH, Kennedy Sh. Prevalence and incidence of chronic pelvic pain in primary care: evidence from a national general practice database. *Br J Obstet Gynecol* 1999;106:1149-1155.

Öst LG. Applied relaxation: description of a coping technique and review of controlled studies. *Behaviour Research and Therapy* 25:397-407.

In: Physical Therapy:
Editor: James P. Bennett

ISBN: 978-1-61122-418-4

Chapter 2

STRESS-RELATED LATENCY IN SENSORY AND AFFECTIVE DIMENSIONS OF REPORTED PAIN IN PATIENTS WITH FIBROMYALGIA SYNDROME

Roger J. Allen and Amy S. Moe
Department of Physical Therapy, University of Puget Sound, Tacoma, WA, United States

ABSTRACT

Patients with fibromyalgia syndrome (FS) experience variable persistent pain, yet causes of episodic pain flares are often inexplicable. Stress has been suggested as a trigger, however reported correlations between pain intensity and same-day stress are low. Several recent FS case studies report notable increases in pain ten days following stressful episodes. This study's purpose was to assess the impact of stress across time on latent pain intensity changes as well as sensory and affective pain responses in a larger FS patient sample. Thirty-eight patients with FS admitted to a four-week multidisciplinary pain program completed the following inventories daily for 4 weeks: Daily Stress Inventory (DSI), Visual Analog Scale (VAS) for pain intensity, McGill Pain Questionnaire Short Form (MPQSF). Affective (MPQSF-A) and sensory (MPQSF-S) pain scores from the MPQSF were analyzed separately. Serial-lag correlations between DSI and VAS, MPQSF-S, and MPQSF-A assessed the impact of daily stress across time on the intensity, sensory, and affect-tive response to episodic pain flares. Since 35 of 38 participants rated the intake/initial evaluation day of the program as the most stressful day of their four week stay in the program, three separate one-way repeated measures ANOVAs were conducted to compare VAS, MGQSF-A, MGQSF-S scores for each day of participation (up to 14 days) following the stressful initial intake day. Pain intensity, sensory, and affective scores yielded very low correlations with same-day stress. However, seria l-lag correlations revealed significant relationships between high stress days and pain flares occurring ten days later for pain intensity (r=+0.53), pain sensation (r=+0.46), and affective responses (r=+0.59). Based on ANOVA with Bonferroni correction, VAS scores yielded significant points at 3, 10, and 13 days following program intake. MGSFQ-S yielded a significant point 10 days following intake. MGSFQ-A yielded signify-cant points at 10 and 13 days following intake. In all statistical comparisons, the most significant mean elevations in pain responses occurred on day 10 following program intake/initial evaluation. It may be concluded that stress increases are associated with delayed episodic pain flares and pronounced sensory and affective responses to pain occurring ten days later in patients with FS.

INTRODUCTION

Fibromyalgia syndrome (FS) is a chronic pain disorder of unknown etiology characterized by widespread pain, hypersensitivity to palpation in at least 11 of 18 specific tender points, sleep disturbances, and fatigue. [1,2,3] Other common but less consistent comorbid clinical manifestations may include lightheadedness, memory loss, insomnia, prolonged morning stiffness, depression, headache, vestibular complaints, esophageal dysmotility, restless legs syndrome, irritable bowel syndrome, interstitial cystitis, and urodynia. [2,4] Diagnosis is based on patient history and physical examination, with 4kg/cm^2 pressure stimulation applied via dolorimetry to assess the presence of tender points. [4,5] Due to "chronic widespread pain" (CWP) patients with this syndrome tend to produce high scores on the McGill Pain Questionnaire [6], with a tendency to select dramatic descriptive adjectives, indicative of a strong affective component to the manner in which they perceive their pain. [4]

This syndrome has been found to be present in all age, ethnic, and cultural groups studied to date. [4] The prevalence of FS is estimated by the American College of Rheumatology to be approximately 2% in the United States population, with 3.5% of women and 0.5% of men manifesting the syndrome. [3] Due to the persistence of pain and unpredictable episodic flares in intensity, as a group, patients with FS have a significantly higher unemployment rate than the population at large. [7] In order to maintain employment, it is estimated that approximately 30% of patients with FS work shorter hours or perform less physically taxing work. [8] Approximately 15% receive disability compensation due to their symptoms. [3]

The term fibromyalgia syndrome was adopted to replace the original "fibrositis" because inflammatory features have not been found to underlie the etiology of the syndrome. [4] Even the present "fibromyalgia" nomenclature is problematic in that it implies involvement of fibrous ("fibro") and muscular tissue ("my"). [4] Given the absence of histological findings supporting a peripheral disease, some views of FS suggested it might be a psychosocial disorder. [4] Approximately 30% to 40% of patients with FS are diagnosed with depression, however, between 40% and 60% do not meet criteria for any current affective or somatoform disorder. [4] While comorbid psychological factors such as depression may be present a purely psychological etiology has now largely been dismissed [2], with the current focus heavily shifting toward investigation of neural mechanisms. [2,4] Curiously, topical anesthesia has been reported to have no effect on tender point pain severity induced by deep pressure stimulation, indicating that any involved neural structures are likely to be rostral to the site of perceived pain. [9] Current pathophysiolgical conceptualizations of FS suggest it is likely a disorder of nociceptive and neuroendocrine dysfunction. [2,4]

Symptoms of FS are chronic and persistent, however, patients with FS often experience episodic pain flares that are frequently inexplicable. [10,11] Many factors have been hypothesized to modulate FS pain or account for changes in episodic pain and the occurrence of painful flares. Some of these include fatigue [11], sleep disturbance or deprivation [12, 13], poor activity pacing [11], cold exposure [11], physical exertion [2], concentrations of neurochemicals such as tryptophan [14] and substance P [4], and the experience of stress. [1,2,3,7,15-18]

It is well documented that people with FS have significantly higher levels of perceived stress than age and gender-matched controls. [7] Accordingly, many authors have alluded to the significance of psychological factors and mood disturbance in the exacerbation of chronic pain [5,19-22], often attributing a dysfunction of the stress response system. [23,24] There are, however, a number of possible relationships between the experience of stress and FS. [25] Stress may be a precipitating factor in the onset of FS, individuals with FS may have altered reactivity to stressors, and/or psychophysiological axes of the stress response may modulate FS pain.

Stress is frequently cited as a potential etiological factor in the development of FS. [26] Many individuals with FS experience high levels of distress [2] and report that their symptoms started following and significant period of physical or emotional stress. [27,28] Buskila and Neumann report that controlled studies have determined that subjects with FS have higher rates of physical or emotional trauma prior to the onset of their symptoms. [20] Clauw lists "stressors" that may be capable of triggering fibromyalgia. These include peripheral pain syndromes, infections, physical trauma, psychological stress/distress, hormonal alterations, drugs, vaccines, and catastrophic events. [2] Curiously, victims of accidents have been found to have higher incidence of FS than those people who cause the accidents, underscoring the notion that our most severe stressors are those over which we have no control or those that are inescapable or unavoidable. [29]

The tender points, essential to the diagnosis of FS, have been chara-cterized by Wolfe as a "sedimentation rate for distress," due to popul-ation-based investigations establishing increased tender point sensitivity in distressed individuals. [30] Recent literature suggests that while tender point reactivity is associated with the experience of stress, the CWP component of fibromyalgia may be only modestly associated with stress. [2] While there is some evidence suggesting a relationship between distress and fibromyalgia development, a specific pathophysiological linkage has yet to be fully established. [31]

The presence of FS may influence response to daily life stressors by lowering positive affect and increasing stress reactivity over time. [32] In comparisons using matched women with osteoarthritis who experienced similar levels of pain, women with FS reported experiencing more inte-rpersonal stress, responded less adaptively to both stressors and chronic illness, and appeared particularly vulnerable to the negative effects of social stress. [32] Studies also show increased rates of post-traumatic stress disorder in patients with FS, affecting approximately 50% of the FS population. [33] Okifuji and Turk observe that living with FS and its related symptoms serves as an ongoing stressor in and of itself and the high level of emotional distress inherent in FS may reflect the struggle of FS patients to adapt to their condition. [1]

The experience of stress as a modulating factor in FS pain has been explored with a variety of approaches with mixed results. Many patients with FS report that both physical and psychological stress exacerbate their symptoms. [3] Studies confirm patients with FS report pain flare-ups that occur hours or even days following either a physically or psychologically stressful event. [34] It has been reported that in one patient sample 65% of FS patients considered stress to be an aggravating factor in their pain and that stress-reducing strategies, such as taking a warm bath or relaxing, were considered ameliorating factors. [1] Bansevicius and colleagues report that following long duration mental stress, increases in FS pain were not associated with increased EMG responses [17], indicating that a more central sensitization model may be responsible for stress-related increases in pain.

Clauw and Williams offer the observation that while stress may influence pain flares, these episodic increases in pain are more likely to be linked to personally relevant events and daily hassles, compared to major catastrophic incidents. [16] Two studies failed to find a worsening of pain symptoms occurring in response to catastrophic events. No difference in pain complaints were noted in New York and New Jersey residents who happened to have been surveyed prior to September 11, 2001 and then just after the terrorist attack on the World Trade Center. [35] A similar finding was published from a sample in Washington D.C., in response to the September 11 Pentagon attack, where patients with FS reported no increase in pain complaints or other symptoms following the attack. [36]

Individuals with FS have been reported to manifest functional abnormalities in multiple pathways of the neuroendocrine stress response, including the sympathoadrenal (SA) system and the hypothalamic-pituitary-adrenal (HPA), hypothalamic-pituitary-thyroid (HPT), and hypothalamic-pituitary-somatotrophin (HPS) axes. [2,4,16,37] Whether each of these stress axes serve as a modulating factor explaining day to day fluctuations of perceived FS pain is not just a matter of the potential psychophysiological mechanism being in place, but the timing of pain changes in relation to when triggering stressors occur. Psychophysiological effects from the SA system have a nearly immediate onset; those from the HPA axis may take minutes to manifest and have response durations of 2-4 hours, whereas the HPT axis takes nearly two weeks to manifest observable symptoms and may persist for weeks. [38-42]

Two investigations took a detailed look at the day-by-day temporal relationship between stress and pain flares in a limited number of patients with FS using multiple case study designs. [15,43] Both studies had patients complete daily stress assessments and multiple pain rating scales for a period of ten weeks. Stress was found to have a very low correlation with same-day perceived pain intensity (r=+0.01-+0.03). [15] However, using serial lag correlations, much stronger relationships were observed between stress on a given day and perceived pain intensity three days later (r=+0.35-+0.40) and ten days later (r=+0.45-+0.70). Similar results were reported regarding a ten day delayed relationship between stress and pain-related function (r=+0.44-+0.54). For all subjects combined 17 out of 19 days that were categorized as moderately or severely stressful resulted in significant pain flares ten days later [15]. The same methodological approach was applied to assess possible daily changes reported by 3 FS patients in dynamic or migrating pain distribution as a result of stress over time. The results were similar, with low correlations between the extent of pain distribution and same-day stress (r=+0.05-+0.16), and stronger correlations with pain experienced three (r=+0.29-+0.34) and ten (r=+0.50-+0.64) days post stress. [43] These findings are consistent with previous results from patients with complex regional pain syndrome, who evidenced the ten-day delay, but not the three-day delay. [44] Similar findings coming from two different patient populations suggest the possibility that there may be a common stress factor operating to provide modulation of pain sensitivity in neuropathic pain that includes a mechanism to delay the onset of pain flares for more than a week.

Since evidence for this delayed pain response in FS patients is based on very small numbers of patients, further investigation of the temporal relationnship between stress and pain in a larger FS sample may prove enlightening.

PURPOSE

The purpose of this study was to assess the impact of stress across time on changes in perceived pain intensity and reported sensory and affective dimensions of pain in patients with fibromyalgia syndrome.

METHOD

Institutional Review Board (IRB) Approval: Given that this study involved a secondary analysis of de-identified data, it was reviewed and granted IRB exempt status by the Department of Physical Therapy's designee of the University of Puget Sound's Institutional Review Board on November 28, 2008.

Participants: Participants contributing data for this study included 38 patients with a diagnosis of FS who had completed a four-week multidisciplinary pain program. For 34 female and 4 male participants the mean age at admission was 44.2 years (range 28-73 years) and mean time since FS diagnosis was 39.9 months (range 4-110 months). Patients attended the clinic Monday through Friday for four weeks, with initial intake on a Friday and no data collection on Saturday or Sunday.

Procedural Overview: This study involved a secondary analysis of de-identified data collected from a private multidisciplinary pain clinic between September 2003 and August 2007. Patients with FS who participated in a four-week pain management program completed daily stress, pain, and anxiety assessments. Pain was evaluated for intensity as well as its sensory and affective components. Serial lag correlations assessed potential delayed temporal relationships between stress and multiple pain dimensions. Initial analysis revealed that 35 of 38 participants rated the intake/initial evaluation day of the program as either the most, or second most, stressful day they experienced during the four-week program. This day was, therefore, utilized as a salient stressful episode marking the starting point for tracking participant pain responses to stress over time in further analyses.

Many patients entering in this program reported leading relatively sedentary lives prior to their participation. The initial intake day required them to participate in a 45 minute physical therapy evaluation, 60 minutes of functional activity and circuit training baseline assessments, 60 minutes of exercise tolerance baseline assessments, 45 minutes of occupational therapy assessment, 60 minutes of activities of daily living and functional tolerance assessments, intake appointments with the attending physician, nursing staff, attending psychologist, a beginning didactic class, and (if indicated) an initial evaluation with a vocational rehabilitation counselor. This day was mentally and physically challenging and represented a major change in the patients' daily life routines, thus meeting Selye's conceptualization of a stressor that calls the body's mechanisms of adaptation into play. [38] The mean Daily Stress Inventory score for this day was 45.5.

Dependent Measures: A summary quantitative rating of the perceived stress experience for each day was determined using the Daily Stress Inventory (DSI) [45], which is a self administered assessment taking into account both the occurrence and impact of daily life stressors. Each of 58 items are rated as to whether or not they occurred that day and, if so, given a Likert scale intensity rating from 1 ("occurred but was not stressful") to 7 ("caused me to panic"). Each patient's daily stress score was a total of the values given to all Likert rated items. Total daily scores in the 0-20 range are indicative of low stress, whereas a highly stressful day is evidenced by a score in the range of 50-80. The DSI has been found to discriminate well between stressful workdays and weekends [45,46] and correlate highly with other summary measures of daily stress. [15,47] Generalizability coefficients indicate that the scale has significant homogeneity and a useful degree of stability. [47]

Pain intensity was quantified using a Visual Analog Scale (VAS) by having patients place a mark on a 10 cm scale to indicate perceived pain intensity, with the extreme right side of the line representing "no pain" and the left extreme end representing "most pain imaginable." The daily pain intensity score was a measurement to 0.1 cm of how far to the left the patient placed a mark on the scale. There is a significant body of research supporting the reliability and validity of the Visual Analog Pain scale as a sensitive measure of both pain intensity and temporal changes in perceived pain. [48,49] It should be noted that two studies have reported that, as straightforward and simple as the instrument appears to be, between 7% and 11% of patients in research samples found it confusing and difficult to complete. [50,51] This underscores the importance of utilizing multiple measures to assess perceived pain, representing diverse parameters of the pain experience.

The McGill Pain Questionnaire Short Form (MPQSF) was employed to assess separately sensory (MPQSF-S) and affective (MPQSF-A) dimensions of perceived pain on a daily basis. [6] Daily scores can range from 0-33 for the sensory subscale and 0-12 for the affective. Numerous studies have supported statistically the reliability, factor structure, and concurrent validity of the McGill Questionnaire. [48,52,53] This questionnaire has been used frequently in the assessment of pain among patients with FS. [4]

Participants completed each assessment every weekday for 4 consecutive weeks during the program. A notable limitation to the use of existing data for secondary analysis in this study was that patients did not complete the assessments on weekend days. With data representing only five consecutive days out of each week, important gaps exist which do not allow a complete temporal assessment of the relationship between stress and pain across time.

Analyses: Serial-lag correlations between DSI and VAS scores and between DSI and MPQSF-S and MPQSF-A scores assessed the impact of daily stress across time on intensity, sensory, and affective dimensions of episodic pain flares. The serial lag correlations utilized repeated Pearson product-moment correlation coefficients to look for associations between stress scores and individual pain measures for stress and pain occurring the same day, then stress with pain scores for the following day (lag = 1 day), then stress with pain two days later (lag = 2 days), with continuous lag correlations up to 14 days. This approach was used to reveal if there were consistent time delays in the appearance of episodic pain flares following a particularly stressful day and has been utilized for this purpose in numerous previous studies. [15,41-44]

Three separate one-way repeated measures ANOVAs were then conducted to compare three dimensions of pain responses via VAS, MGQSF-S, MGQSF-A scores for each day of participation (up to 14 days) following the stressful initial intake day. Post-hoc pairwise comparisons with Bonferonni correction were performed. Since previous studies found evidence for a ten-day delay between the occurrence of salient stressors and a subsequent pain flare, the fourteen-day period for analysis allowed sufficient time to observe whether a similar pattern was evident within this sample. All statistical analyses were conduced using SPSS-PC statistical package, version 14.0.

RESULTS

The first issue to address is the strength of association between stress and same-day pain activity. Pain intensity, sensory, and affective scores were not found to be well correlated with same-day stress, with r values of +0.11, +0.07, and +0.10 respectively. These data indicate that reported stress was not associated with same-day pain intensity or sensory and affective pain responses.

Serial-lag correlations, however, revealed stronger relationships between high stress days and pain flares occurring ten days later for pain intensity (r=+0.53), sensory pain response (r=+0.46) and affective pain response (r=0.59). Table 1 presents serial lag correlations between daily stress ratings and pain responses across all three measures. Although useful for identifying potential temporal delays in pain reactivity due to stress, the serial lag correlations underestimate the specific impact that peak stress days may have on subsequent peak pain episodes, in that the lag correlations included a large number of days that were not rated as stressful which were followed by pain fluctuations due to other factors. In consideration of that potential underestimation, correlations were calculated for the stress rating of only the initial intake day and each of the three pain measures. These yielded strong correlations between intake day and stress for VAS measured pain intensity (r=+0.73), for the sensory pain dimension (r=+0.71), and for affective responses to pain (r=+0.84).

Table 1. Serial lag correlations between daily stress ratings and pain responses measured via VAS (Visual Analog Scale), MPQSF-S (McGill Pain Questionnaire Short Form - Sensory), and MPQSF-A (McGill Pain Questionnaire Short Form - affective).

Lag in Days	VAS	MPQSF-S	MPQSF-A
0	+0.107	+0.069	+0.102
3	+0.311	+0.019	-0.226
4	-0.123	-0.026	+0.117
5	+0.021	+0.118	-0.019
6	+0.001	+0.009	-0.014
7	+0.106	-0.134	+0.097
10	+0.532	+0.464	+0.589
11	+0.287	+0.241	+0.280
12	+0.051	+0.015	+0.109
13	+0.369	+0.273	+0.379
14	+0.074	+0.110	+0.137

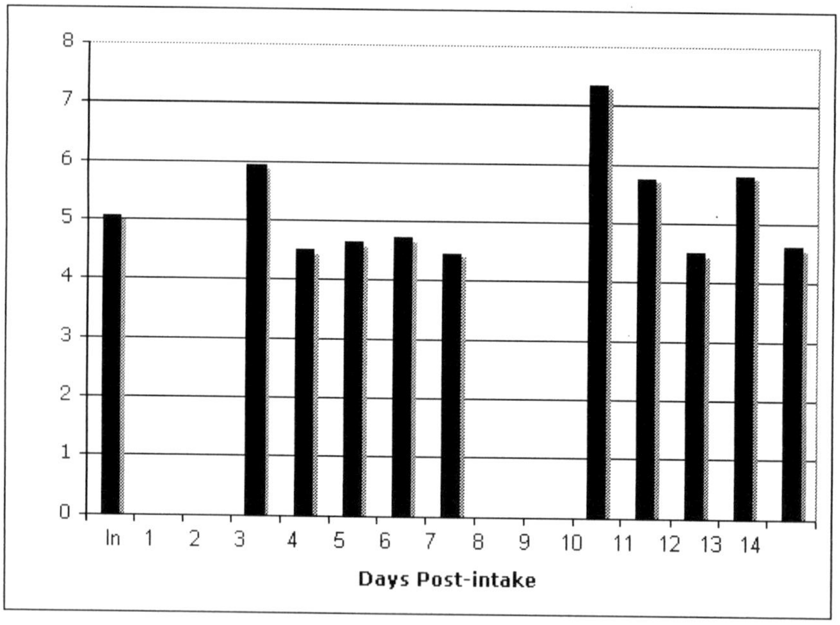

Figure 1. Daily Visual Analog Scale pain intensity mean scores across all patients for 14 days post program intake.

A one-way repeated measures ANOVA on pain intensity scores via VAS was significant (p<0.001). Post-hoc tests with Bonferroni correction revealed day 3 (mean score 5.92/10), day 10 (mean score 7.34/10), and day 13 (mean score 5.81/10) as significantly increased pain ratings. Figure 1 illustrates changes in pain intensity, averaged across all participants, for 14 days following initial intake.

A one-way repeated measures ANOVA was also run on MPQSF-S and revealed significance (p<0.001). Post-hoc tests with Bonferroni correction identified that on day 10 (mean score 14.5/33) subjects had a significantly heightened sensory experience of pain. Figure 2 represents reported sensory pain scores.

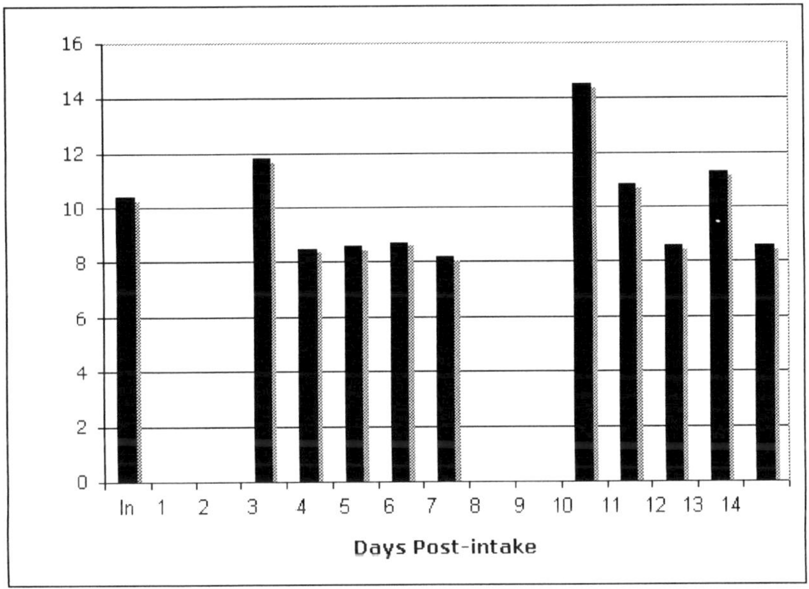

Figure 2. Daily sensory pain mean scores across all patients for 14 days post program intake - derived from McGill Pain Questionnaire Short Form.

Finally, a one-way repeated measures ANOVA was conducted on MPQSF-A and was significant (p<0.001). Post-hoc tests with Bonferroni correction revealed that on day 10 (mean score 3.74/12) and day 13 (mean score 2.42/12) subjects had significantly increased affective experience of pain. Figure 3 illustrates reported affective pain scores over the same 2-week period.

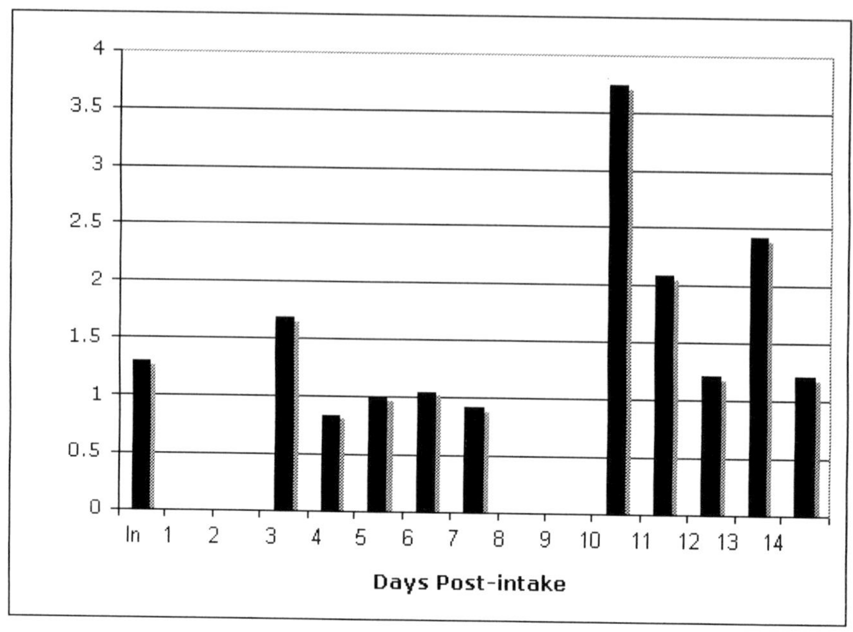

Figure 3. Daily affective impact of pain mean scores across all patients for 14 days post program intake - derived from McGill Pain Questionnaire Short Form.

For all three dimensions of reported pain, note the elevated pain response on day ten following intake. In all comparisons, the most significant mean elevation in pain ratings occurred 10 days following intake. Affective responses were the pain parameter showing the most striking day 10 elevation. Additional significant pain peaks occurred on days 3 and 13 in reference to VAS assessment of pain intensity. While this trend was observed for the other two pain measures, it was found to be significant only for day 13 of the affective response.

While the statistical analyses of group data points to a ten-day delayed stress response, it is clear that not all patients manifested this latent pain reaction. Although not part of the formal analysis, it is interesting to note how many patients showed a definable spike in pain on the tenth day following the initial intake day across the pain parameters measured. Of the 38 patients, 26 had a VAS score on the tenth day in excess of one standard deviation above his/her individual VAS mean, 24 had sensory scores more than one standard deviation above the individual mean, and 29 reported similarly high affective scores. The three patients who did not rate the intake day as particularly stressful were among those who did not register peak pain responses to any of the three pain measures. Depending upon the pain parameter considered, 69%-83% of the 35 patients rating the intake day as notably stressful experienced a pain flare ten days later. Additional information on these patients that might have been evaluated to hypothesize what factor(s) might account for individual differences in the manifestation of latent pain responses was not available in this data set.

Discussion

According to Jones and Clark, subjectively reported patient experiences indicate that flares in FS pain can occur hours even days following either a physically or psychologically stressful event. [34] The findings of this study are consistent with that observation. Significant pain flares following a notably stressful day occurred ten days later, as evidenced by ANOVA comparisons of daily pain responses following the stressful initial intake day and serial-lag correlations comparing stress to resultant pain in a stepwise manner across time, using this sample of 38 patients with FS. The specific timing of these delayed pain responses is also consistent with previous case studies reporting latent pain experiences following definable moments of stress in other patients with FS, which reported delayed pain flares occurring on days three and ten post-stress. [15,43]

The findings of the present study are based on patient self-reports of stress and perceived pain. It must be acknowledged that patient responses in these self-reports may be viewed as one form of pain behavior. Schwartz and colleagues point out that central to behavioral theories of chronic pain is the notion that psychological factors can elicit pain behaviors. Further, they assert that pain behaviors are more likely under conditions of stress. [19] This phenomenon may certainly be a factor underlying some associations between perceived FS pain and stress, however, it cannot account for changes in reported pain perception that occur days after a stressful event has occurred. To understand significantly delayed pain responses we need to search for neuromodulating factors that could potentially include a plausible latency mechanism.

Although the observed three-day delayed spike in VAS measured pain intensity appears to be a unique feature of FS patients' reactions to stress, it is noteworthy that three studies have reported the ten-day delayed pain reaction manifesting itself in patients with CRPS. [41,44,54] This suggests that the mechanism delaying the painful response to stress is not specific to a particular neuropathology. Rather, there is a mechanism with a built-in latency factor that is modulating the ascending pain message or its central neural processing.

Clauw has observed that numerous investigators in the pain field now feel that chronic pain is a "disease" and that many of the underlying etiological factors or modulating mechanisms may be similar. [2] Individuals experiencing chronic pain may have a problem with the sensory processing of pain rather than an abnormality in the region of the body where the pain is perceived. [2] Specifically in relation to FS, Russell asserts that there exists broad experimental support to conceptualize FS as "chronic widespread allodynia." [4] This would suggest, pathophysiologically, that episodic variations in perceived FS pain could be influenced by neuroendocrine modulators operating on either the central or peripheral nervous system. The specific timing of these delayed pain reactions may provide necessary insight into what mechanisms are responsible for the post-stress modulation of pain perception.

The three-day delay in VAS measured pain intensity, which based on available research appears unique to FS, is the most difficult to account for using psychophysiological models of stress. At this point in time, available literature does not offer a psychophysiological axis of the stress response specifically manifesting symptoms three days after the experience of an inciting stressor. It must be pointed out, however, that in this study the aggregate stressful experience of the patients' intake day involved stressors that were both cognitive and physical. As well as requiring a significant change in daily routine and mental adaptation to daunting new challenges, these patients were exposed to a significant amount of unaccustomed physical activity. One hypothesis to account for the observed three-day delay may be the effects of "delayed-onset muscle soreness" (DOMS) [55,56] whose impact may have been heightened by the global allodynia inherent in FS. [4] This phenomenon is reported to appear in normal subjects between 12 and 48 hours following unaccustomed increase in skeletal muscle activity. [55] Due to the fact that pain data in this study were not collected on the Saturday and Sunday following the stressful Friday intake day, the specific 12-48 hour window for observing a DOMS effect was missed, meaning the observation of increased pain 72 hours later may reflect either the trailing end of a DOMS reaction or the manifestation of another pain modulating mechanism.

The initial increased physical activity of the intake day and approximate timing of the three-day pain flare gives a DOMS explanation for this first flare some potential plausibility. This delay was also apparent in the sensory and affective data, but not found to be significant. Close examination of the pain response data also reveals a significant common flare appearing on day thirteen in both pain intensity and affect measures. This is three days after the strong ten-day delayed peak. Given the possibility that the thirteen-day delay may be a latent stress reaction to the salient peak in pain occurring on day ten (the pain peak serving as a new stressor), it may be argued that rather than a DOMS response, there is an unidentified psychophysiological mechanism that is manifesting a type of gradually diminishing reverberation to the initial stressor.

There is a plausible psychophysiological mechanism to account for the ten-day delay observed across all parameters of pain in this investigation and in previous studies involving patients with both FS and CRPS. This mechanism involves the hypothalamic-pituitary-thyroid (HPT) axis. [54] This is a very well established component of the psychophysiological response to stress [38,57-60], yet one that is given relatively little attention in the chronic pain literature compared to the contributions of the HPA axis. [40] An essential feature of this stress pathway is that, following the psychogenic release of thyroxine (T4) and triiodothyronine (T3) from the thyroid gland the thyroid hormones are immediately rendered temporarily inert by serum thyroxine-binding globulins (TBGs). [57] The timing of the half-life of this bond is such that the release of free thyroxine produces a well established symptomatic peak ten days after initial release. [39,61]

The psychophysiological release of thyroid hormones via the HPT axis begins with limbic activation of the paraventricular nucleus of the hypothalamus. Paraventricular neurosecretory cells release thyroid stimulating hormone releasing factor (TRF) into the hypohypophyseal portal system, which in turn carries it to the anterior pituitary. In response to the presence of TRF anterior pituitary basophils release thyroid stimulating hormone (TSH) into systemic circulation. When TSH encounters its target, the thyroid gland, T3 and T4 are released and immediately bound to TBGs to be slowly released with a peak serum concentration of the active hormones occurring approximately ten days later. [38,39,57]

Previous literature has established connections between the activity of thyroid hormones via the HPT axis and the experience of pain. Neeck reports that a likely contributing factor to the dysfunction of the stress response system in FS patients involves alterations in thyroid function. [24] Edmondson and colleagues found that hyperthyroid mice had more sensitivity to pain and showed decreased duration of morphine effectiveness. [62] Allen, McCann, and Hazra monitored daily stress and pain levels and took daily blood draws for microplate assay of bound and free T4 in a patient with CRPS over a ten-week period. They found pain peaks occurring at ten-day intervals following particularly stressful days and observed that each stress-related delayed pain flare was accompanied by a significant elevation in free serum T4. [54]

Chapman points out that the interaction of both sensory and emotional components is integral to the experience of pain. [63] The influence of free thyroxine on pain is to modulate both the magnitude of nociceptive input and central reactivity. [54] By operating on sodium channels to increase excitability of peripheral axons, the presence of thyroxine may increase nociceptor firing delivering the distal pain message to the CNS. Further, via increased reticular system activation, thyroxine increases cerebration, thus potentially heightening anxiety and emotional responses to the incoming pain message. [39] This neuromodulation view is supported by findings of Sorensen and colleagues who report "temporal summation was more pronounced in patients with FM. This is an indication of central sensitization (hyperexcitability)." [64] Also notable for patients with FS, insomnia is an effect of the increased cerebration rate, due to thyroxine. [39] There is consistent evidence in the literature that loss of sleep is an important pain modulating element for patients with FS. [12,13] Thus, even if there is no change in a distal lesion, elevated free serum thyroxine can potentially cause an increase in nociceptive input and altered central processing of the pain message. The painful stimulus is perceived as stronger and independently emotional suffering may be more intense. Both elements are evidenced in the present study via increases in the reported sensory and affective components of pain ten days following stress as assessed by the MPQSF scales, with the strongest effect appearing as a tenth day increase in the affective component of pain.

The psychogenic release of thyroxine via the HPT axis and its subsequent influence on perceived pain, following a ten-day delay, are summarized in Figure 4.

Although there is plausibility for the hypothesis that elevated levels of psychogenically released T4 may be a modulating factor in stress-related FS pain, there are notable reports in the literature that offer an apparent contradictory view to this mechanism. Greenen and colleagues report that some of the symptoms of FS resemble hypothyroidism. [65] In a study of 38 patients with FS, Lowe reports "the percentages of primary and central hypothyroidism in this group of fibromyalgia patients are extremely higher than those for the general population." [66] However, two studies have found that while there is a tendency for FS patients to manifest low basal thyroid hormone levels, they are still within the normal range. [67,68] While patients with FS may tend to have low basal thyroid hormone levels it is still plausible that temporal increases in T3 and T4 may trigger episodic flares. This may be a more pronounced effect in the hypothyroid individual given the possibility of increased neural sensitivity to thyroid hormones, due to chronically low basal levels.

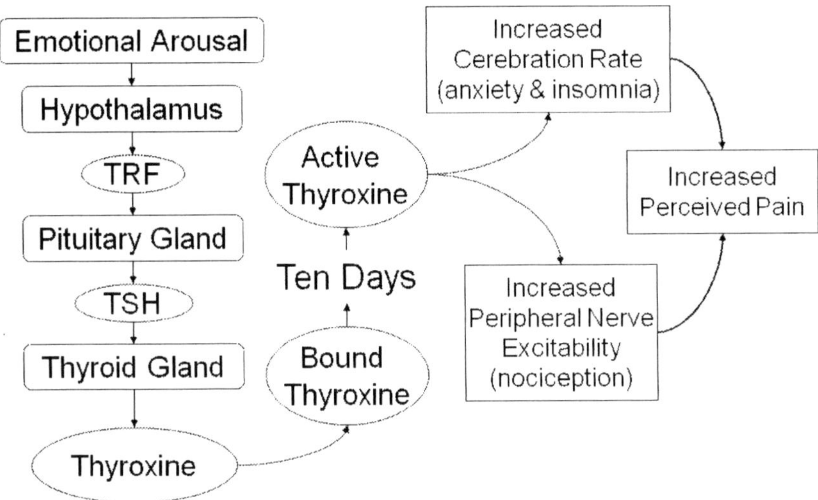

Figure 4. Psychophysiological pathway of thyroxine release due to psychogenic stress and resulting mechanisms of delayed increased pain perception.

A second issue that should be considered pertaining to modulation via the HPT axis has to do with observations that under some stress conditions, stress decreases thyroid hormone release. [38,40] Selye reviewed the diametrically opposed responses of the HPT axis to stress and concluded that whether thyroid hormones increase or decrease appears to be a species and stressor specific phenomenon. [38] In stressed rabbits and horses, thyroid output increases [38,58], whereas it tends to decrease in stressed rats. [58] In human subjects, mild stressors of short duration are typically found to decrease HPT activity, while more intense or chronic stress tends to increase thyroid hormone release. [38] "Stress can either increase or decrease TSH secretion depending upon conditions (intensity and duration of stress, type of stress used) and the animal species examined. In summary, we must conclude that an effect of stress upon thyroid function itself - like its influence on TSH secretion - is definitely demonstrable, but its intensity and direction depend on so many conditioning factors that generalizations are difficult to make." [38] Therefore, even given possible connections between hypothyroidism and FS and the fact that under some conditions HPT axis activity decreased, elevated stress-triggered thyroxine remains a plausible mechanism to account for the 10-day delayed pain response in patients with FS.

The findings from the present study, and similar recent work investigating delayed pain responses following stressful episodes, imply that stress may play a causal role in the precipitation of painful flares occurring ten days later in patients with FS and perhaps other neuropathic pain conditions. There is now sufficient literature regarding this relationship to begin evaluating the adequacy of currently available information for establishing stress as a causal factor in delayed pain responses. Epidemiologically, there are five criteria of judgment for establishing causal relationships. [69] These include strength of the association, consistency of the association, a temporally correct association, specificity of the association, and biological plausibility. [69]

Strength of association refers to the degree to which the element being evaluated as the cause (stress) is related to the occurrence of the effect (increased pain perception). In the present study, correlations between patient ratings of stress and pain perception ten days later ranged from r=+0.46-+0.59 across the three measures of pain. Targeting a specific stressful day and observing pain reactions ten days later yielded correlations from r=+0.71-+0.84. To establish that the relationship is a consistent one requires that the same association also be observed in other circumstances, such as in studies conducted on other patient populations. As previously discussed, this same delayed pain observation has been reported in other studies with FS patients, finding correlations ranging from r=+0.34-+0.60 [15,43], and in studies with CRPS patients that report correlations between r=+0.28-+0.88. [41,44,54] All these studies, however, represent small sample sizes. A temporally correct association means that the cause must precede the effect. Given the nature of observations, analyses, and results, it is clear that the flares in pain being reported occurred after the stressful event. In other words, elevated stress preceded the pain flares, not the reverse. The correct temporal relationship is, therefore, in evidence. Establishing specificity of the association requires that all other plausible explanations for the observed flares in pain be eliminated as potential causal factors, either via experimental control or findings that demonstrate they are not operating as causal components. In this case, as in many others attempting to establish causal connections, all possible additional causes have not been ruled out via controls or other evidence. Biological plausibility requires that there is reasonable evidence for a pathophysiological mechanism accounting for the observed relationship. The effects on pain perception of psychogenically released thyroxine and the ten-day delay in its activation due to TBGs provide a plausible mechanism to account for the specific relationship reported here. [54] In short, there is now evidence to support four of five causality criteria. There is evidence for a strong, consistent, temporally correct, and plausible relationship between stress and delayed pain, with specificity work yet to be done to assess the influence of other potential factors that may account for this phenomenon.

Given the potential value that this delayed pain response finding has to our understanding of mechanisms and potential control of FS pain, further inquiry is warranted. It would be useful for future work, with a more robust patient sample size, to take daily thyroxine assays on patients seamlessly tracked over time for stress and pain changes, using a protocol similar to that used with CRPS patients. [54] Since not all patients in this study experienced a delayed pain response, future studies could utilize comprehensive patient profile information to determine if factors exist that predict whether or not a given patient will manifest delayed pain responses. Considering that this phenomenon has now been observed in both patients with FS and CRPS, investigation into delayed pain responses to stress in patients with other neuropathological conditions would help determine if this mechanism is somehow uniquely influencing the pathophysiology of the conditions already studied, or if it is modulating a general alteration in pain system sensitivity.

In a more general sense, the methodology and findings of the present study underscore how important it is for future studies to precisely observe the timing of salient stressors in relation to changes in perceived pain. Far too many studies in current literature are so vague on this point that stress and pain are assessed as concurrent events, with no consideration given to even the direction of the temporal relationship. Thoughtful research design and observation of time intervals between stress activation and resultant perceived pain changes may add significantly to our understanding of the multifaceted mechanisms of chronic neuropathic pain.

The findings of the present study have immediate implications for patients, therapists, and other medical practitioners working FS patients. It has long been understood that patients suffering from a variety of chronic pain conditions, including FS, frequently experience seemingly random flares in pain intensity. [10] The results of this study suggest that stress may lead to pain flares occurring ten days following the experience of significant stressors. This information may benefit patients by providing an explanation and insight into some previously inexplicable pain increases, differentiating between pain flares brought on by latent reactions to stress versus other actual or imagined triggers, and allowing the ability to predict and plan for future pain flares resulting from stress. These findings may also assist health care providers in timing treatment for patients with FS and facilitating discrimination between pain flares precipitated by therapeutic activity versus those triggered by stress.

Conclusion

The findings of this investigation support observations from case studies indicating that, although there appears little relationship between same-day perceived pain levels and stress, patients with FS experience delayed flares in perceived pain occurring ten days after stressful events. Understanding that these delayed pain responses exist may help account for some previously inexplicable pain episodes, and help both patients and therapists discriminate between stress-related flares and those brought on by activity at home, work, or during therapy.

Acknowledgments

The authors wish to acknowledge and thank Jeffrey Kline, MD, PhD; Chelsea Athing, DPT; Julia Looper, PT, PhD; Casey Pyle, DOS; and Mauri Terao, DPT for their valuable input and contributions to this investigation.

References

[1] Okifuji, A; Turk, DC. Stress and psychophysiological disregulation in patients with fibromyalgia syndrome. *Appl Psychophys and Biof.* 2002; 27(2):129-141.

[2] Clauw, DJ. Fibromyalgia. In: Fishman, SM; Ballantyne, JC; Rathmell, *JP. Bonica's management of pain. 4th ed.* Philadelphia, PA: Lippincott Williams and Wilkins; 2010. 471-488.

[3] Wolfe, F; Smythe, HA; Yunus, MR; Bennett, RM; Bombardier, C, Goldenberg, et al. The American College of Rheumatology 1990 Criteria for the classification of fibromyalgia. Report of the multicenter criteria committee. *Arthritis Rheum.* 1990; 33(2):160-72.

[4] Russell, IJ. Fibromyalgia syndrome. In: In: Loeser, *JD. Bonica's management of pain. 3rd ed.* Philadelphia, PA: Lippincott Williams and Wilkins; 2001. 543-556.

[5] Banks, SM; Kerns, RS. Explaining high rates of depression in chronic pain: a diathesis-stress framework. *Psychol Bull.* 1996;119: 95–110.

[6] Melzack, R. The McGill Pain Questionnaire: major properties and scoring methods. *Pain.* 1975;1: 277-299.

[7] Theadom, A; Copley M. Dysfunctional beliefs, stress and sleep disturbance in fibromyalgia. *Sleep Med.* 2008; 9:376-381.

[8] Wolfe, F; Anderson, J; Harkness, D. Work and disability status of persons with fibromyalgia. *J Rheumatol.* 1997; 24:1171-1178.

[9] Kosek, E; Ekholm, J; Hansson, P. Increased pressure pain sensibility in fibromyalgia patients is located deep to the skin but not restricted to muscle tissue. *Pain.* 1995; 63; 335-339.

[10] Staud, R; Rodriquez, ME. Mechanisms of disease: pain in fibromyalgia syndrome. *Nat Clin Pract Rheumatol.* 2006; 2(2):90-98.

[11] Malt, EA; Olafsson, S; Lund, A; Ursin H. Factors explaining variance in perceived pain in women with fibromyalgia. *BMC Musculoskel Dis.* 2002; 3:12.

[12] Moldofsky, H; Scarisbrick, P; England, R. Musculoskeletal symptoms and non-REM sleep disturbance in patients with "fibrositis syndrome" and healthy subjects. *Psychosom Med.* 1975; 37(4):341-351.

[13] Branco, J; Atalaia, A; Paiva, T. Sleep cycles and alpha-delta sleep in fibromyalgia syndrome. *J Rheumatol.* 1994; 21(6):1113-1117.

[14] Moldofsky, H; Warsh, JJ. Plasma tryptophan and musculoskeletal pain in nonarticular rheumatism ("fibrositis syndrome"). *Pain.* 1978; 5:65-71.

[15] Harlow, LM; Kumiji, KT; Allen, TL; Allen, RJ. Effect of perceived psychogenic stress on pain intensity and timing of increased pain episodes in patients with fibromyalgia syndrome. *J Orthop Sport Phys.* 2005; 35(1):A17.

[16] Clauw, DJ; Williams, DA. Fibromyalgia. In: Mayer, EA; Bushnell, MC. *Functional pain syndromes: presentation and pathophysiology.* Seattle, WA: IASP Press; 2009.

[17] Bansevicius, D; Westgaard, RH, Stiles T. EMG activity and pain development in fibromyalgia patients exposed to mental stress of long duration. *Scan J Rheumatol.* 2001;30:92-98.

[18] Dailey, PA; Bishop, GD; Russell, J; Ellen, FM. Psychological stress and the fibrositis/fibromyalgia syndrome. *J Rheumatol.* 1990;17:1380-1385.

[19] Schwartz, L; Slater, MA; Birchler, GR. Interpersonal stress and pain behaviors in patients with chronic pain. *J Consult Clin Psych.* 1994; 64:861–864.

[20] Buskila, D; Neumann L. Musculoskeletal injury as a trigger for fibromyalgia/posttraumatic fibromyalgia. *Curr Rheumatol Rep.* 2000; 2:104-108.

[21] Turk, DC; Swanson, KS; Wilson, HD. Psychological aspects of pain. In: Fishman, SM; Ballantyne, JC; Rathmell, *JP. Bonica's management of pain. 4th ed.* Philadelphia, PA: Lippincott Williams and Wilkins; 2010. 74-85.

[22] Chapman, CR; Turner, JA. Psychological aspects of pain. In: Loeser, JD. *Bonica's management of pain. 3rd ed.* Philadelphia, PA: Lippincott Williams and Wilkins; 2001. 180-191.

[23] Martinez-Lavin M. Stress, the stress response system, and fibromyalgia. *Arthrit Res Ther.* 2007;9(4):216-223.

[24] Neeck, G. Pathogenic mechanisms of fibromyalgia. *Ageing Res Rev.* 2002;1(2):243-255.

[25] Van Houdendove, B; Egle, U; Luyten, P. The role of stress in fibromyalgia. *Curr Rheum Rep.* 2005;7(5):365-370.

[26] Goodman, CC; Fuller, KS. *Pathology: implications for the physical therapist. 3rd ed.* St. Louise, MO. Saunders. 2009.

[27] Clauw, DJ; Chrousos, GP. Chronic pain and fatigue syndromes: Overlapping clinical and neuroendocrine features and potential pathogenic mechanisms. *Neuroimmunomodulat.* 1997;4(3);134-153.

[28] Turk, DC; Okifuji, A; Starz, TW; Sinclair, JD. Effects of type of symptom onset on psychological distress and disability in fibromyalgia syndrome patients. *Pain.* 1996; 68:423-430.

[29] Chrousos, GP; Gold, PW. The concepts of stress and stress system disorders: overview of physical and behavioral homeostasis. *JAMA.* 1992;267(9):1244-1252.

[30] Wolfe, F. The relationship between tender points and fibromyalgia symptom variables: evidence that fibromyalgia is not a discrete disorder in the clinic. *Ann Rheum Dis.* 1997;56(4):268-271.

[31] McClean, SA; Clauw DJ. Predicting chronic symptoms after an acute "stressor" - lessons learned from 3 medical conditions. *Med Hypotheses.* 2004;63(4):653-658.

[32] Davis, MC; Zautra, AJ; Reich, JW. Vulnerability to stress among women in chronic pain from fibromyalgia and osteoarthritis. *Ann Behav Med.* 2008;23(3):215–226.

[33] Cohen, H; Neumann, L; Haiman, Y; Matar, MA; Press, J; Buskila, D. Prevalence of post-traumatic stress disorder in fibromyalgia patients: overlapping syndromes or post-traumatic fibromyalgia syndrome? *Semin Arthritis Rheum*. 2002;32:38-50.

[34] Jones, KD; Clark, SR. Individualizing the exercise prescription for persons with fibromyalgia. *Rheum Dis Clin N Am*. 2002;28:419-436.

[35] Raphael, KG; Natelson, BH, Janal, MN. A community-based survey of fibromyalgia-like pain complaints following the World Trade Center terrorist attacks. *Pain*. 2002;100(1-2):131-139.

[36] Williams, DA; Brown, SC; Clauw DJ. Self-reported symptoms before and after September 11 in patients with fibromyalgia. *JAMA*. 2003; 289(13):1637-1638.

[37] Crawford, LJ; Pillemer, SR; Kalogeras, KT. Hypothalamic-pituitary-adrenal axis perturbations in patients with fibromyalgia. *Arthritis Rheum*. 1994;37:1583-1592.

[38] Selye, H. *Stress in health and disease*. Boston, MA: Butterworths; 1976.

[39] Guyton, AC; Hall, JE. *Textbook of medical physiology*. 10th ed. Philadelphia, PA: Saunders; 2000.

[40] Helmreich, DL; Parfitt, DB; Lu, XY; Akil, H; Watson, SJ. Relation between the hypothalamic-pituitary-thyroid (HPT) axis and the hypothalamic-pituitary-adrenal (HPA) axis during repeated stress. *Neuroendocrinol*. 2005;81:183-192.

[41] Allen, RJ; Hulten, JM; Roelofson, MJ; Martin, TG; McCormack; SA. Delayed pain reactions due to stress in patients with complex regional pain syndrome. *Physiother*. 2007;93:S293.

[42] Allen RJ. New discoveries into the symptom patterns of peripheral neuropathies and neuropathic pain. *Physical Therapy 2006: Annual Conference & Exposition of the American Physical Therapy Association*. Orlando, FL, June 23, 2006.

[43] Allen, RJ; Bittenbender, CJ; Smith, AK; Townson, KB; Blankenship, SA. Delayed episodic pain reactions due to perceived psychogenic stress in patients with fibromyalgia syndrome: Case series. *J Rehabil Med*. 2008;47:92.

[44] Hulten, JM; Martin, TG; McCormick, SA; Roelofsen, MJ; Allen, RJ. Influence of perceived stress on delayed onset pain episodes and related functional changes in complex regional pain syndrome patients. *Neurol Rep*. 2002;26(4):190-191.

[45] Brantley, PJ. The Daily Stress Inventory. Odessa, FL. *Psychological Assessment Resources*. 1989.

[46] Brantley, PJ; Cocke, TB; Jones, GN; Goreczny, AJ. The Daily Stress Inventory: validity and the effect of repeated administration. *J Psychopathol Behav.* 1988;10(1):75-81.

[47] Brantley, PJ; Waggoner, CD, Jones, GN; Rappaport, NB. A daily stress inventory: development, reliability, and validity. *J Behav Med.* 1987;10(1):61-73.

[48] Chapman, CR; Syrjala, KL. Measurement of pain. In: Loeser, JD. *Bonica's management of pain. 3rd ed.* Philadelphia, PA: Lippincott Williams and Wilkins; 2001. 310-328.

[49] Ohnhaus, EE; Adler, R. Methodological problems in the measurement of pain: a comparison between the Verbal Rating Scale and the Visual Analog Scale. *Pain.* 1975;1:379-384.

[50] Kreemer, EF; Atkinson, JH; Ignelzi, RJ. Measurement of pain: patient preference does not compound pain measurement. *Pain.* 1981;10:241-248.

[51] Revill, SI; Robinson, JO; Rosen, M. The reliability of a linear analog for evaluating pain. *Anesthesia.* 1976;31:1191-1198.

[52] Chapman, CR; Casey, KL; Dubner, R. Pain measurement: an overview. *Pain.* 1985 ;22:1-31.

[53] Syrjala; KL; Chapman, CR. Measurement of clinical pain: a review and integration of research findings. In: Benedetti, C; Chapman, CR, Moricca, G; eds. *Advances in pain research and therapy.* Vol 7. New York: Raven; 1984. 71-101.

[54] Allen, RJ; McCann, CJ; Hazra, SV. Relationship between delayed episodic pain flares and release of the stress-related hormone thyroxine in a patient with complex regional pain syndrome. *J Orthop Sport Phys.* 2009; 39(1):A70-71.

[55] Cerny, F; Burton, H. Exercise physiology for health care professionals. Campaign, IL: *Human Kinetics*; 2004.

[56] Lieber, RL; Friden, J. Morphologic and mechanical basis of delayed-onset muscle soreness. *J Am Acad Orthop Surg.* 2002;10:67-73.

[57] Mason, J; Southwick, S; Yehuda, R. Elevation of serum free triiodothyronine, total triiodothyronine, thyroxine-binding globulin, and total thyroxine levels in combat-related posttraumatic stress disorder. *Arch Gen Psychiatry.* 1994 ;51:629-41.

[58] Furr, MO; Murray, MJ; Ferguson, DC. The effects of stress on gastric ulceration, T3, T4, reverse T3 and cortisol in neonatal foals. *Equine Vet J.* 1992;24(1):37-40.

[59] Farmer, C; Dubrevil, P; Couture, Y; Brazeau, P; Petitclerc, D. Hormonal changes following an acute stress in control and somatostatin-immunized pigs. *Domest Anim Endocrinol.* 1991;8(4):527-36.

[60] Schell, E; Theorell, R; Hasson, D; Arnetz, B; Saraste, H. Stress biomarkers associations to pain in the neck, shoulder and back in healthy media workers: 12-month prospective follow-up. *Eur Spine J.* 2008; 17:393-405.

[61] Sander, PJ. Endocrine dysfunction concurrent with fibromyalgia. In: Ostalecki, S. *Fibromyalgia: The complete guide from medical experts and patients*. Sudbury, MA: Jones and Bartlett Publishers; 2008. 83-84.

[62] Edmondson, EA; Bonnet, KA; Friedhoff, AJ. The effect of hyperthyroidism on opiate receptor binding & pain sensitivity. *Life Sci.* 1990; 47(24):2283-2289.

[63] Chapman, CR. The psychophysiology of pain. In: Fishman, SM; Ballantyne, JC; Rathmell, *JP. Bonica's management of pain. 4th ed.* Philade-lphia, PA: Lippincott Williams and Wilkins; 2010. 375-387.

[64] Sorensen, J; Graven-Nielsen, T; Henriksson, KF; Bengtsson, M; Arendt-Nielsen, L. Hyperexcitability in fibromyalgia. *J Rheumatol.* 1998;25:152-155

[65] Greenen, R; Jacobs, JWG; Bijlsma, JWJ. Evaluation and management of endocrine dysfunction in fibromyalgia. *Rheum Dis Clin N Am.* 2002; (28):389-404.

[66] Lowe, JC. Thyroid status of 38 fibromyalgia patients: implications for the etiology of fibromyalgia. *Clin Bull of Myofasc Ther.* 1997;2(1):47-64

[67] Riedel, W; Layka, H; Neeck, G. Secretory pattern of GH, TSH, thyroid hormones, ACTH, cortisol, FSH, and LH in patients with fibromyalgia syndrome following systemic injection of the relevant hypothalamic-releasing hormones. *Z Rheumatol.* 1998;57(supp 2):81-87.

[68] Neeck, G; Riedel, W. Thyroid function in patients with fibromyalgia syndrome. *J Rheumatol.* 1992;19:1120-1122.

[69] Kramer, S; Dramer, S. *Mausner and Bahn Epidemiology*. Philadelphia, PA: W.B. Saunders; 1985.

In: Physical Therapy
Editor: James P. Bennett

ISBN: 978-1-61122-418-4

Chapter 3

Breathing Pattern Disorders in Physical Therapy: A Musculoskeletal Perspective

T. Clifton-Smith and J. Bartley
The Auckland Regional Pain Service, Auckland District Health Board, Auckland, New Zealand

Abstract

While body norms such as body temperature, heart rate and blood pressure, and lung volumes are routinely measured by health practitioners, breathing patterns are usually overlooked. Breathing pattern refers not only to lung function and respiration, but also to biomechanics and motor control. In particular, clinical observations of rate and depth of breaths per minute, and patterns of breathing - i.e. nose versus mouth and upper chest versus the energy efficient diaphragm. However, it is important to note that there is so much more to breathing in and out than a nose/diaphragm pattern in the treatment and assessment of breathing pattern disorders. Breathing is one of our most vital functions and a disordered breathing pattern can be the first sign that all is not well, whether it be biomechanically, physiologically or psychologically. For example: breathing rapidly sharply reduces blood carbon dioxide levels. The shift in carbon dioxide chemistry (hypocapnia) may cause physiological changes in the body leading to muscle fatigue, spasm (tetany) and pain.

Breathing pattern disorders affect people of all ages and stages in the population, and appear in all areas of clinical practice. They cause widespread distress and anxiety to the individual, their families and friends, as well as causing high costs to communities in days lost from school or work, and to the healthcare system itself. Physiotherapeutic strategies have been used since the early 1960's in the treatment of breathing pattern disorders in both people with organic lung disease and those without. Cardiorespiratory physiotherapy is well established within the orthodox medical literature - assessment and treatment regimes contain components of breathing education and retraining.

The focus of this chapter will be on the emerging area of musculoskeletal physiotherapy and breathing pattern disorders. Physiotherapists are ideally placed to recognise and treat these disorders, both within the public health and private healthcare systems.

INTRODUCTION

Physiotherapy treatment regimes have been involved in rehabilitation for over a century. The specialty area of respiratory physiotherapy has evolved over time and is well established in orthodox health practice [1]. The first literature referring to breathing pattern disorders and breathing re-education within the physiotherapy profession was in 1960's in the cardiorespiratory speciality area [2,3]. Physiotherapeutic strategies have been used since the early 1960's in the treatment of Breathing Pattern Disorders in both people with organic lung disease and those without [4-10].

Current cardiorespiratory physiotherapy practice focuses on assessment and treatment of patients with organic lung disorders, patients with neuromuscular disorders, pre and post surgical care and intensive care, non medical treatment of patients with respiratory disease and pulmonary rehabilitation. All have components of breathing education [9-12]. Breathing Pattern Disorders are fast becoming recognised within the speciality area of musculoskeletal and sports physiotherapy [13] and private practice [1]. Whilst still having a significant role in the more likely areas of lung disease and of anxiety, the focus of this chapter will be the emerging area of musculoskeletal physical therapy. Breathing patterns not only reflect the functioning of the respiratory system but also that of the biomechanical system as well as the cognitive state. It is essential therefore, that physiotherapists from all specialty areas consider the assessment and treatment of a patient's breathing pattern.

Breathing plays a key role in the neuro-musculo-skeletal system. Breathing correctly assists posture, spinal stabilisation [14], cardiovascular and lymphatic flows, abdominal and bowel movements [15], leading to physiological and physical health and vitality. Poor breathing patterns quickly can disrupt the homeostasis in the body leading to an array of disorders including musculoskeletal problems [16,17]. Chaitow, Bradley & Gilbert [18] state "Nowhere in the body is the axiom of structure governing function more apparent than in its relation to respiration. Ultimately, the self-perpetuating cycle of functional change - creating structural modification - leading to reinforced dysfunctional tendencies can become complete, from whichever direction dysfunction arrives."

WHAT IS A BREATHING PATTERN DISORDER?

Breathing Pattern Disorders appear to be simple, yet they are complex not only by historical definition but also in aetiology and treatment regimen. The orthodox medical literature has attempted to define breathing pattern disorders and hyperventilation [19]. A clear definition of what constitutes a Breathing Pattern Disorder is an evolving process, and various disciplines are providing unique perspectives which, when combined, give a multi-dimensional understanding of the multi-faceted function that is breathing [4,20,21]. In the view of the authors both disorders exist as separate entities with the suggestion hyperventilation can occur as an extreme form either chronically or acutely in conjunction with a breathing pattern disorder. A current working definition has been postulated within the physiotherapy literature; 'Inappropriate breathing which is persistent enough to cause symptoms, with no apparent organic cause' [22]. This is the favoured definition of the authors from the view point that it encompasses hyperventilation and breathing pattern disorders and can encompass acute and chronic episodes. It is important to note that symptoms may not interrupt daily life, but may impact on specific tasks - e.g. elite athletes and their performance. If an athlete has an inefficient breathing pattern when partaking in their activity/ sport this may cause premature breathlessness or lower limb fatigue that is non reflective of cardiovascular fitness or any organic pathology. Consider the patient with neck or shoulder pain who is not responding to treatment as predicted; inefficient breathing patterns lead to increased respiratory accessory muscle activation and increased work of breathing all of which can add to musculo-skeletal issues, such as a shoulder or neck problems.

What Triggers a Disorder?

The cause is believed to be compensation for physiological, bio-mechanical, and psychological triggers. An extensive list of factors thought to trigger disordered breathing (Table 1) [4,20,23-27]. However once the pattern is established the breathing pattern disorder becomes habituated and can exist as an entity of its own or exist alongside the trigger.

Breathing Physiology

Respiratory Control

Breathing is controlled mainly by a "breathing centre" in the brain stem, which is involved in the homeostatic regulation of oxygen (O_2) and carbon dioxide (CO_2) levels in the body [28]. Reflex control of breathing relies principally on cerebral spinal fluid CO_2 levels [28]. Physiologically every cell in the body requires O_2 to survive, yet the body's need to rid itself of CO_2 is the most important stimulus for breathing in a healthy person. It is the most potent chemical affecting respiration [29]. The limbic system in our brain, which coordinates the "fight-or-flight" response can unconsciously override the normal homeostatic regulation of CO_2 levels in the body [30] as can our conscious brain or neocortex [28]. This predominantly occurs in situations of acute stress or in emergencies. The normal partial pressure of CO_2 (pCO_2) in the lung alveoli and arterial blood is 40mm Hg with 35–45mm Hg considered the normal range [28]. Hypocapnia occurs when the arterial pCO_2 level drops below 35mm Hg.

What Happens When CO_2 Levels Goes Down?

At rest, humans were designed to breathe slowly, predominantly using their diaphragms. The average breathing rate for adults is 10-14 breaths per minute [28,31]. However due to a multitude of triggers (Table 1) our pattern can alter and habituate.

Table 1. Aetiological Factors in Breathing Pattern Disorders.

Biomechanical factors
Postural maladaptations
Upper limb movement
Chronic mouth breathing
Cultural, for example, 'tummy in, chest out', tight waisted clothing
Congenital
Overuse, misuse or abuse of musculo-skeletal system
Abnormal movement patterns
Braced posture, for example, post-operative
Occupational, for example, divers, singers, swimmers, dancers, musicians
Physiological / Biochemical factors
Lung Disease
Metabolic Disorders
Allergies- Post-nasal drip, rhinitis, sinusitis
Diet
Exaggerated response to decreased CO_2
Drugs, including recreational drugs, caffeine, aspirin, alcohol
Hormonal, including progesterone
Exercise
Speech/laughter
Chronic low grade fever
Heat
Humidity/ Heat
Altitude
Psychological factors
Anxiety
Stress
Panic disorders
Personality traits, including perfectionist, high achiever, obsessive
Suppressed emotions, for example anger
Conditioning/learnt response
Action projection/anticipation
History of abuse
Mental tasks involving sustained concentration
Sustained boredom
Pain
Depression
Phobic avoidance
Fear of symptoms/Misattribution of symptoms

Physiologically a mismatch occurs between the pattern of breathing and metabolic demand, especially at rest. The respiratory rate and minute volume (the volume of air inhaled and exhaled per minute) may increase and this leads to a hyperventilation state where, by definition, the increase in minute volume exceeds the metabolic demands for O_2 and arterial pCO_2 is lowered [32,33].

For example, it has been shown that computer work can lead to breath holding, particularly on the inspiratory breath [32]. Breath holding increases the work of the accessory respiratory muscles, sternocleidomastoid and scalene muscles shorten, the head protrudes, breathing is now predominately apical (upper chest), inhalation exceeds exhalation and the body becomes saturated with O_2. The body thinks it is exercising or responding to stress or a temporary threat, CO_2 is flushed away faster than it is produced, as no physical activity/ movement is occurring. The result is a rise in the pH of blood, extracellular fluid and cerebrospinal fluid, making the body more alkaline [33].

Respiratory Alkalosis

Acute alkalosis increases central nervous system arousal and skeletal muscle activation all necessary for an acute "fight-or-flight" response facilitating the ability to detect and escape from danger more readily. Ironically this same 'fight-or-flight" response when prolonged can contribute to musculoskeletal disorders [34]. These consequences are discussed later. Respiratory alkalosis also affects hemoglobin uptake of O_2, coronary artery and cerebral blood flow [35].

A Chain Reaction Occurs at a Cellular Level.

Lowering arterial pCO_2 induces an acute respiratory alkalosis and CO_2 moves from intracellular to extracellular fluids. This lowering of CO_2 levels creates many physiological changes but of particular relevance to the musculoskeletal system are:

a) threshold alteration to sensory and motor axons which causes depolarisation or excitation of the nerve motor unit
b) smooth muscle constriction and
c) altered O_2 uptake secondary to the Bohr Effect [17,33].

The increase in pH enhances the likelihood of motor unit nerve depolarisation or excitation [17,33] contributing to an increased central nervous system arousal. The increase in pH also improves muscle function as seen in short duration cycle sprints [36] contributing to the increased skeletal muscle activity again necessary in a "fight-or-flight" response. Increased central nervous system arousal and increased skeletal muscle activation meant that one was more likely to escape from acute danger. If prolonged, over stimulation, fatigue and ultimately increased sensitisation can become problematic.

When pH increases, smooth muscles in vessels in the gut and bronchi constrict [37]. Tissue oxygenation is reduced due to vasoconstriction and inhibition of O2 transfer from haemoglobin; i.e. respiratory alkalosis increases the affinity of haemoglobin (Bohr Effect), so that haemoglobin binds tightly to O2 reducing O2 delivery to tissue cells. This can explain the concept of muscle aching at low levels of effort [3].

The discovery of smooth muscle cells in collagen can potentially explain the presentation of increased muscular and fascial tension amongst individuals with breathing pattern disorders. This implies breathing disorders will play a part in fascial/connective tissue sites - ligaments, menisci, and spinal discs [38-40]. It has even been suggested that perhaps in the hypermobile individual the altered breathing pattern exists as a means to increase tone and stability via the effect of respiratory alkalosis on contractile smooth muscle cells [41]. A rise in pH also causes a systemic arterial vasoconstriction, decreasing global and regional O_2 supply further reducing tissue O_2 delivery [42].

Reduced Muscle Oxygenation

An increase in pH causes a leftward shift of the oxy-haemoglobin dissociation curve reducing local tissue O_2 supply (Bohr effect) [28]. The increased neural excitation associated with the central nervous system arousal contributes to increased muscle tension and muscle spasm [17]. If the increased neural excitation, vasoconstriction and reduced tissue oxygen supply occur during sustained, repetitive work this could also contribute to the development of work-related musculoskeletal disorders [43].

Prolonged hyperventilation also influences the alkaloid buffering system [30]. In chronic respiratory alkalosis renal compensatory mechanisms excrete HCO_3^- in order to return the plasma pH back toward the normal range [28,44]. The systemic loss of bicarbonate from intracellular and extracellular fluids reduces the body's ability to buffer any build up of metabolic byproducts such as lactic acid in muscle tissue [30,32]. In this situation skeletal muscle fatigues more readily [30]. In an alkalotic state, muscle lactic acid also increases leading to an increase in blood lactic acid levels [45]. Lactic acid contributes to muscle pain [46].

Biomechanics

Under quiet breathing conditions, the diaphragm accounts for 70-80% of the work of breathing [28]. The neck and shoulder muscles - the scalene, sternocleidomastoid, external intercostals and parasternal intercostal muscles are responsible for the other 20-30% [28].

The Diaphragm

The diaphragm divides the chest cavity, containing the lungs, from the abdominal cavity, containing the abdominal organs. The diaphragm is classically described as consisting of three parts:

- A central tendinous portion
- A muscular portion attached to the ribs
- A muscular portion called crurae attached to the lower spine

Muscle fibres radiate outward and downward from the central tendinous portion to insert in lower parts of the rib cage these muscles form the muscular rib portion of the diaphragm. The muscular portion extending downwards attaching to the lumbar vertebrae are called crurae (Figure 1). Upon inspiration, the diaphragm contracts and descends. This pump-like motion creates a partial vacuum, which draws air into the lungs creating ideal intra abdominal pressures. Breathing predominately into the abdomen is best termed "abdominal breathing". Traditionally this type of breathing has been called diaphragmatic breathing. Good abdominal muscular tone also has a role in efficient diaphragmatic breathing. When the diaphragm contracts and shortens it pushes down against the contents of the abdomen. If the abdominal muscles, particularly transversus abdominis are weak the diaphragm travels downwards against minimal resistance [16]. The diaphragm has the ability to perform the duel role of respiration plus postural stability during movement [14,47]. When all systems are challenged breathing will remain as the final driving force [48].

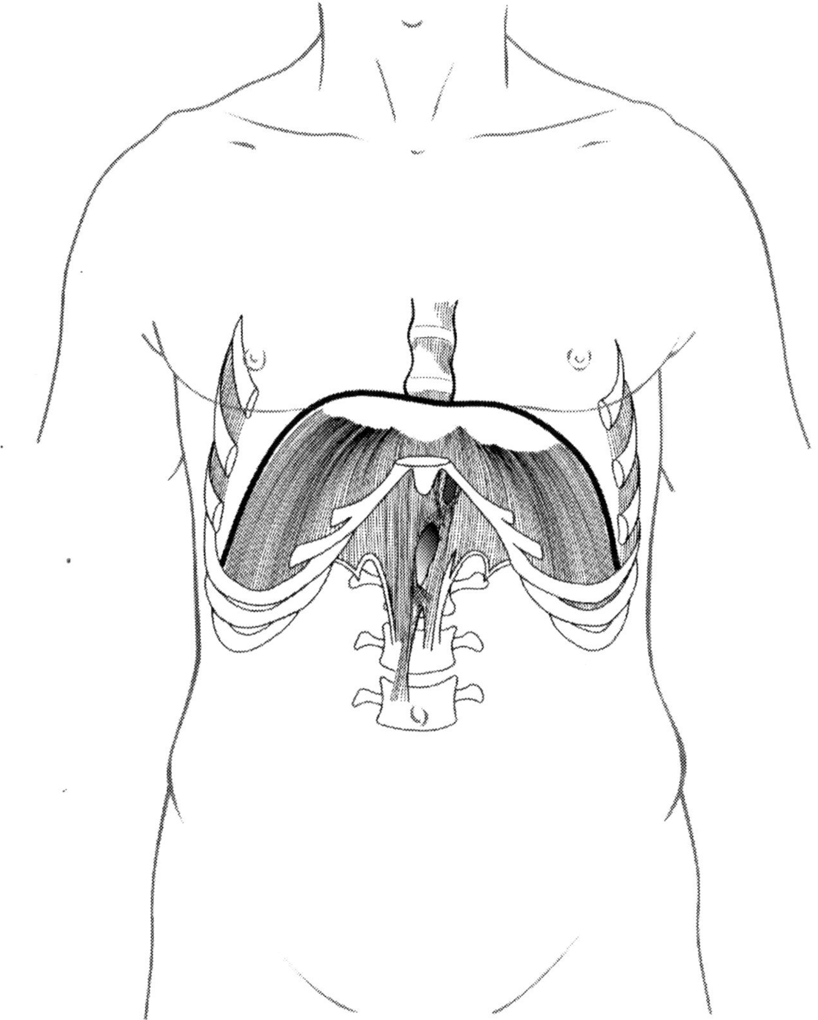

Figure 1. The Diaphragm[26].

Psoas and Quadratus Lumborum

Psoas and quadratus lumborum share a fascial connection to the diaphragm at the lumbar vertebrae, making them vulnerable to disuse, weakness, and myofascial trigger points when diaphragmatic breathing is not observed [49].

The Abdominal Muscles

The abdominal muscles, particularly transversus abdominis, have important roles both in respiration and posture [50]. Good abdominal muscle tone helps the diaphragm work efficiently as well as providing low back support. The abdominal muscles are active during both inhalation and exhalation complementing the action of the diaphragm. Abdominal muscle weakness places increased demands on the other inspiratory muscles. Together with the diaphragm, transversus abdominis, multifidius and the pelvic floor muscles work in unison to establish intraabdominal pressure. All structures add to stability and allow efficient respiration, movement and continence control. Should there be a deviation away from this recruitment pattern i.e. oblique muscle firing first then pressure, ventilation volumes and ultimately the work of breathing is affected [47]. Structural stability is challenged - low back problems and weak pelvic floor muscles are common in poor breathers [50].

Neck and Shoulder Muscles

Many of the muscles of the head and neck attach to the rib cage. These muscles either stabilize or expand the rib cage surrounding the chest cavity during breathing. Normally the diaphragm initiates quiet breathing and other muscles come into play as the breathing cycle continues. There is considerable debate as to the role and relative contributions of each muscle during breathing. Important accessory muscles of respiration include; sternocleidomastoid, scalene muscles, intercostal muscles pectoralis minor and major, trapezius, levator scapulae and serratus anterior [51].

Scalenes

The scalenes are active with each breath, increasing in use with high demands. These are important accessory breathing muscles [52]. Scalenus anterior stabilizes the upper chest during quiet breathing. When overused this results in elevation of the first rib, which can produce thoracic outlet syndrome disorders. With resulting overuse compression from elevation of the first rib can occur in various sites affecting one or all of the following structures: the brachial plexus nerves, the subclavian artery or vein. This can cause a tingling sensation in the fifth and fourth fingers (an ulna nerve distribution) as well as muscle weakness in the hand [52].

Sternocleidomastoid

Problems in these muscles can lead to referred facial and head pain. This muscle plays a role in awareness of body position in space proprioception so dizziness, vertigo (sensation of spinning), nausea and vomiting can occur. With prolonged intense stress this muscle can become overly sensitive creating problems from jaw pain to vertigo [53]. This muscle attaches from behind the ear into the top of the rib cage. When it shortens to elevate the chest, it also pulls the headdownwards and forwards [53]. In this situation the scalene and parasternal intercostal muscles also flex the neck. Because the eyes need to keep looking forward, the head extends at the atlanto-occipital joint and the suboccipital muscles at the base of the skull contract, to extend the head [16]. A typical side posture seen side on, in patients who breathe in their upper chest is of head protrusion.

The Intercostal Muscles

The muscles between the ribs are divided into two groups – the internal and external intercostal muscles. They crisscross each other at right angles. Many patients who have poor breathing patterns overuse these muscles to elevate the ribs. The muscles between the ribs or the costocartilage itself can become quite tender - Tietze syndrome or costochondritis can occur [54].

Upper Trapezius

During good breathing this muscle is at rest, during upper chest breathing this muscle is activated [55,56].

Pectoralis Major and Minor

The pectoralis minor muscle lies deep to pectoralis major. The pectoralis minor muscles attach the ribs to the shoulder blades. During active breathing the pectoralis minor muscles lift the ribs, enlarging the chest cavity and drawing air in. At the same time pectoralis minor lifts the chest upwards, the shoulders are pulled forwards and downwards [16,56]. Overuse of this muscle frequently leads to a tender area just below the outer part of the collarbone where the pectoralis minor muscle attaches to the coracoid process of the scapula. During vigorous breathing, when pectoralis minor contracts this immediately challenges the stability of the scapula - the upper trapezii and the levator scapulae muscles contract to counteract this force [56]. With time and overuse, shoulder protraction, elevation and internal rotation can occur. These chest muscles commonly get tight, causing shoulders to turn inwards, resulting in ineffective breathing patterns.

Serratus Anterior

Serratus anterior deserves a mention; clinically upon presentation of long term breathing pattern disorders this muscle can become compromised. The main function of the serratus anterior is to protract and rotate the scapula, keeping it closely opposed to the thoracic wall and optimizing the position of the glenoid for maximum efficiency for upper extremity motion. If pectoralis minor, upper trapezius and the respiratory accessory muscles shorten serratus anterior can lengthen. Idiopathic winging may appear and glenohumeral movement is compromised; nerve entrapments may occur [57].

What Happens When Breathing Changes?

When breathing changes are maintained for long periods, the ratio of muscular use also alters. The neck and shoulder muscles (backup muscles) start to play an increased role - very soon taking over the lead role and easily becoming the preferred muscles to breathe with which leads to mechanically inefficient postures. In upper chest breathing, inspiratory muscles, such as the sterno-cleidomastoid muscles (which lift the sternum upwards), the scalene muscles (which lift the first two ribs) and the upper trapezii muscles are activated [58,59]. Patients with neck pain commonly have faulty breathing patterns [60]. Breathing problems also predict the development of low back pain [50]. People with back pain brace with their superficial abdominal muscles and diaphragm and have poor core muscle activation [50,61,62]. An awaren-ess of faulty breathing patterns coupled with breathing re-education can provide health professionals valuable, additional tools to help patients with their musculoskeletal disorders [63].

A sequence of changes soon starts to take place - one of the most common is:

- Decreased diaphragm movement
- Loss of lower rib movement
- Pelvic floor weakness,
- Abdominal and spinal muscles imbalance
- Fascial restriction - from the neck to the diaphragm
- Rib movement loss
- Rigid cervical spine (neck)
- Thoracic spine rigidity (mid back) leading to nerve disturbance
- Accessory muscle overuse [64].

What Does This Mean?

- Loss of diaphragm movement sets up a sequence of events leading to inefficient breathing patterns. This also leads to loss of micro massaging to all internal organs, loss of lower oesophageal sphincter tone leading to reflux and gastrointestinal problems and loss of the fluid pump to the cardiovascular system and lymphatic systems leading to venous pooling in the legs.
- Lower rib loss of movement leads to loss of movement of the spinal column resulting in rigidity, stiffness and ultimately pain.
- Pelvic floor weakness leading to bladder problems and a weak base to spinal stabilisers
- Fascial restriction leading to poor postures with structural and ligament immobility
- Spinal rigidity - pain and autonomic nerve disturbance which controls our bodily functions
- 2nd rib loss of movement - decreased lymphatic & blood circulation
- Accessory muscle overuse – lactic acid build up ---loss of efficient blood supply, fatigability of muscles---pain—stiffness--- rigidity---shortened muscles–postural changes---nerve entrapment [65].

Musculoskeletal Implications

Upper chest breathing brings the upper body muscles into play with secondary consequences. The pectoralis major, pectoralis minor, levator scapulae and trapezius muscles are not typically considered accessory respiretory muscles, but all these muscles influence the rib cage and act as extrathoracic anchoring points. Because of their insertions they assist with inspiration, pulling the rib cage up and out. The scalene muscles become more active, lifting and expanding the rib cage during inspiration. The sternocleidomastoid muscles because of their insertion onto the mastoid process and occipital bone, also rotate the back of the head downward. These lifting muscles can create additional stabilising demand from the posterior neck muscles as well as drawing the head and neck forward during upper chest breathing [53].

In chronic upper chest breathing these muscles then have the potential to become overused leading to muscle pain and other associated symptoms. Typical problems include headaches (from tight suboccipital muscles), neck and shoulder pain, chest pain (pectoralis muscles) and low back pain. Until the breathing pattern is corrected, these muscles will continue to be painful.

The Athlete and Sport

Most of the research surrounding sport and breathing has been focused on ventilation and lung capacity. However emerging research supports the benefits of breathing patterns with motor co-ordination plus specific training of the respiratory muscles - inspiratory muscle training (IMT) [66-68]. The work of breathing during maximal exercise can result in changes in locomotor muscle blood flow, cardiac output and both whole-body and active limb oxygen uptake [69]. Evidence suggests the existence of a metaboreflex, with its origin in the respiratory muscles [70]. It is believed this reflex can modulate limb perfusion via stimulation of sympathetic nervous system vasoconstrictor neurons [71]. The fundamental goal of this reflex is the protection of oxygen delivery to the respiratory muscles, thus ensuring the ability to maintain pulmonary ventilation, proper regulation of arterial blood gases and pH and overall organismic homeostasis. This concept has been refered to as blood stealing - a novel idea that literally the muscles of respiration steal oxygen rich blood from the lower limbs [72]. If the muscles of respiration are under undue load this reflex will be triggered long before the athlete meets their cardiovascular capacity.

Ground breaking research was conducted using physiotherapeutic techniques on the effect of breathing pattern retraining on performance in competitive cyclists. Results showed that four weeks of specific breathing pattern retraining enhanced endurance performance, incremental peak power and positively affected breathing pattern and perceived exertion [13]. Not only has research been carried out favouring breathing retraining for performance as above but also showing the importance of diaphragmatic breathing post exhaustive exercise in reducing oxidative stress [73]. Such results indicate breathing retraining should be considered an effective practice to significantly contrast the free radical-mediated oxidative damage induced by intense exercise [74]. Therefore, similar to the way that antioxidant supplementation has been integrated into athletic training programs, diaphragmatic breathing or other meditation techniques could be integrated into many sports as a method to improve performance and accelerate recovery.

Muscle Pain

Muscle pain can be produced by both peripheral and central mechanisms. Peripheral muscle pain is produced by the sensitization of specific pain receptors called nociceptors. Nociceptors are activated by trauma, mechanical overloading and inflammatory mediators such as bradykinin, prostaglandins, adenosine triphosphate (ATP) and protons (H^+)[75]. An acidic tissue pH, which would be aggravated by a loss of systemic bicarbonate and increased lactic acid production, is probably one of the main activators of peripheral nociceptors [45]. Mechanical factors such as poor posture, which leaves some muscles in shortened positions and others under chronic tension in a lengthened position for prolonged periods, as well as muscle spasm can lead to trigger point development in these muscles [46].

The resulting drop in tissue pH would sensitize nociceptors [45]. Systemic factors that compromise muscle and neural energy metabolism are also thought to be contributory [76]. Sensitization of muscle nocioceptive endings leads to the release of the neuropeptides substance P and calcitonin gene related peptide. These peptides created local oedema by dilating local blood vessels and increasing their permeability. The sensitisation of muscle nociceptors is assumed to be the peripheral mechanism leading to muscle tenderness [45]. The influx of nervous impulses from muscle nociceptors into the spinal cord can also lead to central processing changes of pain signals at a dorsal horn level. This leads to a long lasting increase in excitability (central sensitization) due to the effect of glutamate on NMDA (N-methyl-D-aspartate) receptors. This is a possible mechanism for referred muscle pain, a contributory factor to increased peripheral muscle tenderness as well as an explanation for myofascial trigger points [45].

Therefore the muscle pain seen in association with breathing disorders may be secondary to the interplay of a number of factors:

- postural changes associated which place some muscles in shortened positions and others under chronic tension in a lengthened position for prolonged periods would be a factor in muscle trigger point and pain development [46]
- Increased neural excitation associated with respiratory alkalosis contributing to increased muscle tension and muscle spasm [32}
- reduced muscle oxygenation secondary to vasoconstriction and the Bohr Effect
- the systemic loss of bicarbonate compromising the body's ability to buffer the build up of metabolic byproducts such as lactic acid in muscle tissue leading to muscle fatigue [30,32], and muscle pain [45].
- Prolonged peripheral pain leading to changes in pain processing at a central level [45].

Psychological

Psychological factors both influence and are influenced by breathing patterns [77]. It has been suggested that breathing should be examined as an independent variable affecting the psychological process [77]. Some authors, for example, believe it is the fear of the dyspnoea that plays a major factor in panic attacks [78]. It is often the sensation of dyspnoea or muscle discomfort that will limit performance. Anxiety is the commonest factor thought to influence breathing, and it has been noted to cause increased inspiratory flow rate, breathing to become faster and shallower, and/or involving breath holding [77,79]. A number of papers have documented the relationship between stress and respiratory function [80,81]. Similar changes are seen with anticipatory anxiety [82].

Under situations of stress people often hyperventilate adopting a rapid, shallow, predominantly upper chest pattern of breathing. As seen such patterns can lead to a cascade of biomechanical and physiological changes. Acutely, this can apply to performance anxiety [83]. It has been shown that when baseball players performing in intense situations were educated in good breathing techniques they improved more in batting when compared to a sports psychology intervention group [84].

BREATHING RETRAINING

In the medical literature there are many references to abnormal breathing and disease. This presumes that a criterion has been established for what is "normal". Many medical professions base their clinical practice on the principles of "normal" breathing rates and patterns. Disparities are apparent. Key aspects in the physiotherapy literature appear to have the following basic principles in common - education, reassurance, and breathing retraining [2-6,26,85,86].

1. Education on the disorder
2. Self observation of one's own breathing pattern
3. Restoration to a basic physiological breathing pattern: relaxed, rhythmical nose – abdominal breathing.
4. Appropriate tidal volume
5. Education of stress and tension in the body
6. Posture
7. Breathing with movement and activity
8. Clothing Awareness
9. Breathing & Speech
10. Breathing & Nutrition
11. Breathing & Sleep
12. Breathing through an acute episode

The terms breathing exercises, breathing retraining and breathing pattern training are all used in the physiotherapy literature. For the purposes of this chapter assessment and treatment interventions will not be discussed in detail.

Conclusion

Faulty breathing patterns present differently, depending on the individual. Some patients are more inclined to mental distress, fear, anxiety and co-existing loss of self-confidence. Others may exhibit musculoskeletal and more physical symptoms such as neck and shoulder problems, chronic pain and fatigue, poor motor performance. Many are a combination of both mental and physical factors [87].

As a profession our diversity is an asset. The key points of breathing pattern disorders are common to who ever we treat. Expertise is in individual cases whether it is the child with asthma or the elite athlete. The diversity of our profession enables us to approach breathing pattern disorders from different perspectives, yet allows us a cohesive informed approach, as physiotherapy aims to treat the whole person not just the system.

Acknowledgments

The authors would like to acknowledge the contributions and influence of Dinah Bradley and Dr Robert Fried to their work.

Further Reading

Bartley, J; Clifton-Smith, T. *Breathing Matters*. Auckland: Random House; 2006.

URL: *http://www.breathingmatters.com*

References

[1] Nicholls, D; Walton, JA; Price K. *Making breathing your business: enterprising practices at the margins of orthodoxy*. Sage Publications 2009; 13: 333 –356.

[2] Innocenti D. Chronic Hyperventilation syndrome. In P.A. Downey (Ed.) *Cash's textbook of chest, heart, and vascular disorders for physic-otherapists*. 4th ed. London: Faber & Faber; 1987.

[3] Cluff, R. Chronic hyperventilation and its treatment by physiotherapy. *J R Soc Med* 1984; 77: 855-862.

[4] Bradley, D. Physiotherapy breathing rehabilitation strategies. In: Chaitow L, Bradley D, Gilbert C (Eds.). *Multidisciplinary Approaches to Breathing Pattern Disorders*. Edinburgh: Churchill Livingstone; 2002 pp173-195.

[5] Singh, J. Management of hyperventilation. *ACPRC Journal* 2001; 34, 50-5.

[6] Rowbottom, I. The physiotherapy management of chronic hyperv-entilation syndrome. *ACPRC Journal*.1992; 21, 9-12

[7] Thompson, B. Asthma and your child. Christchurch: Pegasus; 1967.

[8] Massery, M. Referred by the Cystic Fibrosis Clinic's PT: Treatment of Posture and Pain. *Pediatric Pulmonology*, Supplement. 2008; 31: 112-114.

[9] Hough, A. *Physiotherapy in respiratory care: An evidence based approach to respiratory and cardiac management* .3rd ed. Glouster: Nelson Thornes Ltd.; 2001.

[10] Gosselink, R. Breathing techniques in patients with chronic obstructive pulmonary disease (COPD). *Chron Resp Dis* 2004; 1: 163 - 172.

[11] Bott, J; Blumenthal, S; Buxton, M; Ellum, S; Falconer, C; Garrod, R; Harvey, A; Hughes, T; Lincoln, M; Mikelsons, C; Potter, C; Pryor, J; Rimington, L; Sinfield, F; Thompson, C; Vaughn, P; White, J; British Thoracic Society Physiotherapy Guideline Development Group. Guidelines for the physiotherapy management of the adult, medical, spontaneously breathing patient. *Thorax* 2009; 64: Suppl1:i1-52.

[12] Kant, S; Singh, G. *Breathing Exercises as adjunct in the management of COPD:* An Overview. Lung India 2006; 23: 165-169.

[13] Vickery, R. The effect of breathing pattern retraining on performance in competitive cyclists, 2007. Available from URL: *http://repositoryaut.lconz.ac.nz/handle/10292/83*.

[14] Hodges, PW; Butler, JE; McKenzie, D; Gandevia, SC. Contraction of the human diaphragm during postural adjustments. *J Physiol* (Lond) 1997; 505: 239-248.

[15] Williams, P (Ed). *Gray's Anatomy* (38th edition). Edinburgh: Churchill Livingstone; 1995.

[16] Hruska, J. Influences of dysfunctional respiratory mechanics on orofacial pain. *Dent Clin North Am* 1997; 41: 211-27.

[17] Schleifer, LM; Ley, R. End-tidal PCO2 as an index of psychological activity during VDT data- entry work and relaxation. *Ergonomics*, 1994; 37:245-54.

[18] Chaitow, L; Bradley, D; Gilbert, C. *Multidisciplinary Approaches to Breathing Pattern Disorders*. London: Churchill Livingstone; 2002.

[19] Molema, J; Folgering, H. *Introduction in abstracts of papers presented at the 3rd International Society of the Advancement of Respiratory Psychophysiology* (ISARP).

[20] Chaitow, L. Biomechanical influences on breathing. In Multidisciplinary approaches to breathing pattern disorders. In: Chaitow L, Bradley D, Gilbert, C (Eds.). *Multidisciplinary Approaches to Breathing Pattern Disorders*. Edinburgh: Churchill Livingstone; pp.83-110.

[21] Gilbert, C. Clinical applications of breathing regulation. Beyond anxiety management. *Behav Modif* 2003; 27: 692-709.

[22] Rowley J. *The role of asthma, stress and posture as aetiological factors in breathing pattern disorders*. 2002 (unpublished)

[23] Gardner, W. The pathophysiology of hyperventilation disorders. *Chest* 1996; 109: 516-535.

[24] Lum, C. Hyperventilation and anxiety state. *J R Soc Med* 1981; 74: 1-4.

[25] Newton, E. Hyperventilation Syndrome, 1997. Available from URL: *http://www.emedicine.com/emerg/topic270.htm*

[26] Bartley, J; Clifton-Smith, T. *Breathing Matters*. Auckland: Random House; 2006.

[27] Burgess, J; Kovalchick, D; Kyes, KB; Thompson, JN; Barnhart S. Hyperventilation following a large-scale hazardous-materials incident. *Int J Occup Environ Health* 1999; 5: 194-7.

[28] West, JB. *Respiratory physiology: the essentials*. Lippincott Williams and Wilkins, Philadelphia 2000.

[29] Marieb, E. *Human Anatomy & Physiology* (5th ed). Harlow: Addison Wesley Longman; 2001.

[30] Von Schéele, BH; von Schéele, IA. The measurement of respiratory and metabolic parameters of patients and controls before and after incremental exercise on bicycle: supporting the effort syndrome hypothesis? *Appl Psychophysiol Biofeedback* 1999; 24: 167-77.

[31] Celli, B. The diaphragm and respiratory muscles. *Chest Surg Clin N Am* 1998; 8: 207-24.

[32] Schleifer, LM; Ley, AR; Spalding, TW. A hyperventilation theory of job stress and musculoskeletal disorders. *Am J Ind Med* 2002; 41: 420-432.

[33] Laffey, JG; Kavanagh, BP. Hypocapnia. *N Engl J Med* 2002; 347: 43-53.

[34] Jacobs, GD. The physiology of mind-body interactions: the stress response and the relaxation response. *Journal Altern Complement Med* 2001; 7 (Suppl 1): S83-92.

[35] Kazmaier, S; Weyland. A; Buhre, W; Stephan, H; Rieke, H; Filoda, K; Sonntag, H. Effects of Respiratory Alkalosis and Acidosis on Myocardial Blood Flow and Metabolism in Patients with Coronary Artery Disease. *Anesthesiology* 1998; 89: 831-837.

[36] Bishop, D; Edge, J; Davis, C; Goodman, C. Induced metabolic alkalosis affects muscle metabolism and repeated-sprint ability. *Med Sci Sports Exerc* 2004; 36: 807-13.

[37] Nixon, PGF; Andrews, J. A study of anaerobic threshold in chronic fatigue syndrome (CFS). *Biol Psychology* 1996; 43: 264.

[38] Schleip, R; Naylor, IL; Ursu, D et al. Passive muscle stiffness may be influenced by active contractility of intramuscular connective tissue. *Med Hypotheses*. 2006; 66:66-71.

[39] Staubesand, J; Li, Y. *Zum Feinbau der Fascia cruris mit besonderer. Berücksichtigung epi- und intrafaszialer Nerven. Manuelle Medizin.* 1996; 34: 196-200.

[40] Yahia, LH; Pigeon, P; DesRosiers, EA. Viscoelastic properties of the human lumbodorsal fascia. *J Biomed Eng* 1993; 15: 425-429.

[41] Chaitow, L. Breathing pattern disorders, motor control, and low back pain *J Osteopath Med* 2004; 7: 34-41.

[42] Guzman, JA; Kruse, JA. Gut mucosal-arterial PCO_2 gradient as an indicator of splanchnic perfusion during systemic hypo- and hyprcapnia. *Crit Care Med* 1999; 27: 2760-5.

[43] Carayon, P; Smith, MJ; Haims, MC. Work organization, job stress, and work-related musculoskeletal disorders. Hum Factors. 1999; 41: 644-63.

[44] Foster, GT; Vaziri, ND; Sassoon, CS. Respiratory alkalosis. *Respir Care* 2001; 46: 384-91.

[45] Mense, S. Muscle pain: mechanisms and clinical significance. *Dtch Ärztebl Int* 2008; 105: 214-9.

[46] Simons, DG; Travell, JG; Simons, LS. *Travell & Simons Myofascial pain and dysfunction: the trigger point manual* (2nd ed.) Philadelphia: Williams and Wilkins; 1999; pp 19-20.

[47] Hodges P, Gandevia S. Activation of the human diaphragm during a repetitive postural task. *J Physiol* (Lond) 2000; 522:165-175.

[48] Hodges P, McKenzie D, Heijnen I, Gandevia S. Reduced contribution of the diaphragm to postural control in patients with severe chronic airflow limitation. *In Proceedings of the Thoracic Society of Australia and New Zealand, Melbourne, Australia*: 2000.
[49] Simons, DG; Travell, JG; Simons, LS. Travell & Simons *Myofascial pain and dysfunction: the trigger point manual (2nd ed.) Philadelphia:* Williams and Wilkins; 1999; p869.
[50] Smith, MD; Russell, A; Hodges, PW. Do incontinence, breathing difficulties, and gastrointestinal symptoms increase the risk of future back pain? *J Pain* 2009; 10: 876-86.
[51] Simons, DG; Travell, JG; Simons, LS. *Travell & Simons Myofascial pain and dysfunction: the trigger point manual (2nd ed.) Philadelphia*: Williams and Wilkins; 1999; p 874.
[52] Simons, DG; Travell, JG; Simons, LS. *Travell & Simons Myofascial pain and dysfunction: the trigger point manual (2nd ed.) Philadelphia:* Williams and Wilkins; 1999; pp 509-10. .
[53] Simons, DG; Travell, JG; Simons, LS. *Travell & Simons Myofascial pain and dysfunction: the trigger point manual (2nd ed.) Philadelphia*: Williams and Wilkins; 1999; pp 308-13. .
[54] Simons, DG; Travell, JG; Simons, LS. *Travell & Simons Myofascial pain and dysfunction: the trigger point manual (2nd ed.) Philadelphia:* Williams and Wilkins; 1999; pp 878.
[55] Mercer, S. Surface Electrode Placement and Upper Trapezius. *Advances in Physiotherapy* 2002; 4: 50-3.
[56] Simons, DG; Travell, JG; Simons, LS. *Travell & Simons Myofascial pain and dysfunction: the trigger point manual (2nd ed.) Philadelphia:* Williams and Wilkins; 1999; pp 846.
[57] Warner, JJ; Navarro, RA. Serratus anterior dysfunction. Recognition and treatment. *Clin Orthop Relat Res*. 1998; 349: 139-148.
[58] Falla, D. Unravelling the complexity of muscle impairment in chronic neck pain. Man Ther 2004; 9: 125–133.
[59] Nederhand, M; Ijzerman, M; Hermens, H; Baten, C; Zilvold, G. Cervical muscle dysfunction in the chronic whiplash associated disorder grade II (WAD-II). *Spine* 2000; 25: 1938-43.
[60] Perri, M; Halford, E. Pain and faulty breathing: a pilot study. *J Bodyw Mov Ther* 2008, 4: 297–306.
[61] Radebold, A; Cholewicki, J; Polzhofer, B; Greene, H. Impaired postural control of the lumbar spine is associated with delayed muscle response

times in patients with chronic idiopathic low back pain. *Spine* 2001; 26; 724-30.

[62] Hodges, P; Richardson, C. Altered trunk muscle recruitment in people with low back pain with upper limb movement at different speeds. *Arch Phys Med Rehabil* 1999; 80: 1005-12.

[63] McLaughlin, L. Breathing evaluation and retraining in manual therapy. *J Bodyw Mov Ther* 2009; 13: 276–282.

[64] Garland, W. Somatic changes in hyperventilating subjects. *Presentation to the International Society for Advancement of Respiratory Psychophysiology congress*, France, 1994.

[65] Clifton-Smith, T. *Breathe to Succeed in All Aspects of Your Life.* Ringwood: Penguin New Zealand, 1999.

[66] Volianitis, S; McConnell, AK; Koutedakis, Y; McNaughton, L; Backx, K; Jones, DA. Inspiratory muscle training Improves rowing performance. Inspiratory Muscle Training Improves Rowing Performance. *Journal of Sports Sciences* 2000; 18: 551.

[67] Volianitis, S; McConnell, AK; Koutedakis, Y; McNaughton, L; Backx, K; Jones, DA. The influence of inspiratory muscle training upon rowing performance in competitive rowers. *Med. Sci. Sports Exerc* 2001; 33: 803-809.

[68] Romer, LM; McConnell, AK; Jones, DA. Inspiratory muscle fatigue in trained cyclists: effects of inspiratory muscle training. *Med Sci Sports Exerc* 2002; 34: 785-792.

[69] Harms, CA; Wetter, TJ; McClaran, SR; Pegelow, DF; Nickele, GA; Nelson, WB; Hanson, P; Dempsey JA. Effects of respiratory muscle work on cardiac output and its distribution during maximal exercise. *J Appl Physiol* 1998; 85: 609–618.

[70] Sheel, AW; Derchak, PA: Morgan, BJ; Pegelow, DF: Jaques, AJ: Dempsey, JA. Fatiguing inspiratory work causes reflex reduction in resting leg blood flow in humans. *J Physiol* 2001; 537: 277-289.

[71] St Croix, CM; Morgan, BJ; Wetter, TJ; Dempsey, JA. Fatiguing inspiratory muscle work causes reflex sympathetic activation in humans. *J Physiol* 2000; 529: 493–504.

[72] McConnell, A. Inspiratory muscle training as an ergogenic aid: credible at last? *Physiology News* 2007, 68.

[73] Martarelli, D; Cocchioni, M: Scuri, S; Pompei, P. *Diaphragmatic Breathing Reduces Exercise-induced Oxidative Stress: Evid Based Complement Alternat Med.* 2009 Oct 29 [Epub ahead of print].

[74] Phillips. M; Cataneo, RN; Greenberg, J; Grodman, R; Gunawardena, R; Naidu, A. Effect of oxygen on breath markers of oxidative stress. *Eur Respir J* 2003; 21: 48–51.

[75] Galloway, SD; Maughan, RJ. The effects of induced alkalosis on the metabolic response to prolonged exercise in humans. *Eur J Appl Physiol Occup Physiol* 1996; 74: 384-9.

[76] Simons, DG; Travell, JG; Simons, LS. *Travell & Simons Myofascial pain and dysfunction: the trigger point manual, (2nd ed.) Philadelphia:* Williams and Wilkins; 1999; pp178-235..

[77] Ley, R. The modification of breathing behaviour: Pavlovian and operant control in emotion and cognition. *Behav Modif* 1999; 23: 441-79.

[78] Ley, R. Panic disorder and agrophobia: Fear of the fear or fear of the symptoms produced by hyperventilation? *J Behav Ther Exp Psychiatry* 1997; 18: 305-16

[79] Umezawa, A. Facilitation and inhibition of breathing during changes of emotion. In: Huruki ,Y; Homma, I; Umezaw, A; Masaoka, Y. (Eds). *Respiration and Emotion.* New York: Springer-Verlag; 2001; pp139-147.

[80] Jack, S; Rossiter, HB; Pearson, MG; Ward, SA; Warburton, CJ; Whipp, BJ. Ventilatory responses to inhaled carbon dioxide, hypoxia, and exercise in idiopathic hyperventilation. *Am J Respir Crit Care Med* 2004; 170: 118-125.

[81] Hodges, PW; Gandevia, S. Changes in intra-abdominal pressure during postural and respiratory activation of the human diaphragm. *J Appl Physiol* 2000; 89: 967-976.

[82] Masaoka, Y; Homma, I. Anxiety and respiratory patterns: their relationship during mental stress and physical load. *Int J Psychophysiol* 1997; 27: 153-159.

[83] Ley, R; Yelich, G. Fractional end-tidal CO2 as an index of the effects of stress on math performance and verbal memory of test-anxious adolescents. *Biol Psychol* 1998; 49: 83-94.

[84] Strack, B: Gevirtz, RN; Sime, W. Effect of heart rate variability biofeedback on batting performance in baseball. *Appl Psychophysiol Biofeedback* 2005; 29: 299

[85] Holloway, EA. The Role of the Physiotherapist in the treatment of Hyperventilation. In B. H. Timmons & R. Ley (Eds.) *Behavioural and psychological approaches to breathing disorders*. New York: Plenum Press; 1994.

[86] Thomas, M; McKinley, RK; Freeman, E; Foy, C; Prodger, P; Price, D. Breathing retraining for dysfunctional breathing in asthma: a randomised controlled trial. *Thorax* 2003; 58:110–115.

[87] Bradley, D; Clifton-Smith, T. *BradCliff® Manual. Writers inc.*, Auckland 2009.

In: Physical Therapy
Editor: James P. Bennett
ISBN: 978-1-61122-418-4

Chapter 4

SHOULDER REHABILITATION: IS THERE A ROLE FOR HOME THERAPY?

Patrick St. Pierre and Mark Frankle
Foundation for Orthopaedic Research (FORE), Tampa, Florida, USA

ABSTRACT

Formal post-operative physical therapy is the standard of care following shoulder surgeries to include arthroscopic reconstructions, decompressions, rotator cuff repairs, and arthroplasties. A significant amount of health care resources are spent on these rehabilitation programs, however their cost-effectiveness and necessity have not been established.

A retrospective analysis conducted of 2 consecutive groups of patients undergoing total shoulder arthroplasty (TSA) for primary osteoarthritis is reviewed. One group was treated with formal physical therapy (PT), and one group was treated with home-based, physician-guided PT. ASES and Simple Shoulder Test (SST) scores significantly improved in both groups at all follow-up periods. Forward flexion and abduction were significantly improved in the home-based group at all time points, whereas an initial improvement in forward flexion and abduction in the formal PT group was lost at final follow-up. There were no significant differences in final ASES or SST scores between groups at final follow-up. However, forward flexion, abduction, and the Short Form-36 physical component summary scores in the home-based group were significantly better than those patients with formal PT at final follow-up. No significant improvements in internal rotation or SF-36 mental component summary were seen within or between the groups at final follow-up. Overall, there was no difference in patient satisfaction.

A home-based, physician-guided therapy program may provide adequate rehabilitation after TSA, allowing for a reduction in cost for the total procedure. Based on these results, we have developed home therapy programs for shoulder surgeries to include arthroscopic procedures in addition to arthroplasties. By focusing on patient-oriented, home-based therapy programs, we allow patients to take full responsibility for their recovery and not rely on an outside agency to be responsible for their result. Based on our early results we suggest this approach works well for many patients, however, supervised PT may still be required for patients who are not progressing as expected. Close physician follow-up and referral to formal PT may be necessary for patients who are not able to meet rehabilitation guidelines on their own. Better collaboration between PT and surgeons can lead to better clinical outcomes, but further studies with valid evaluation of outcome data are necessary.

INTRODUCTION

The number of shoulder surgeries performed by Orthopaedic surgeons has increased markedly over the past two to three decades. Much of this has been to dramatic advancements in arthroscopic procedures, allowing for surgeries previously done as open procedures to be performed with a much less invasive technique.[55] Early results lagged that of their open counterparts, but as these techniques improved, the results have become increasingly equivocal and arthroscopic rotator cuff repair and arthroscopic shoulder reconstructions have become the norm and the preferred technique by many shoulder surgeons [14,42,54,55] As the population ages, osteoarthritis of the glenohumeral joint is a frequent source of shoulder pain and dysfunction. Total shoulder arthroplasty (TSA) is an effective treatment for relieving pain and improving function. [2, 3, 4, 5, 6, 16, 17, 18, 22, 23, 24, 25, 30, 32, 33, 41, 43, 45, 46, 50, 51, 57, 58, 59, 60, 61, 64] Initially, a surgery performed only at "shoulder institutions" and infrequently in the community, the increased number of patients and refinement of techniques has allowed the community Orthopaedic surgeon to take on these surgeries. Finally, the development of the reverse total shoulder arthroplasty (r-TSA) for the treatment of rotator cuff arthropathy has added a successful surgery for a previously very difficult diagnosis. [9, 28] As Orthopaedic surgeons become more adept at this procedure, it is anticipated that the number of these procedures will grow at a substantial rate. With the exception of instability surgery, the final motion and function achieved following all of these surgeries is typically improved compared with preoperative motion. However, the reported improvement in range of motion (ROM) postoperatively is quite variable, and may be related to both preoperative and postoperative factors. [2, 7, 15, 21, 31, 36, 39, 47]

One factor that may influence final function and patient satisfaction is the postoperative rehabilitation protocol. As with other surgeries, patients undergoing shoulder surgery rely on postoperative physical therapy (PT) to regain motion and strength after surgery. Most PT protocols follow a logical progression that begins with gentle, passive mobilization, advances to active motion, and ultimately incorporates muscle strengthening. [7, 10, 12, 35, 37, 65] This progressive PT must carefully balance the need for adequate soft tissue healing while preventing postoperative stiffness. If the postoperative PT program is too protective, stiffness may become a problem. [34] Conversely, an aggressive PT program could jeopardize the integrity of the subscapularis repair and compromise stability and function. Unfortunately, there is a paucity of information in the literature addressing therapy after shoulder surgery. Published clinical series include a variety of rehabilitation protocols, ranging from home therapy programs with minimal therapist direction to fully supervised physical therapy programs. [7, 10, 12, 35, 37, 38, 65]

To our knowledge, only one study has directly compared home versus formal rehabilitation protocols after TSA, and this study demonstrated favorable results after TSA with a home based rehabilitation program. This study was generated out of concern for subscapularis dysfunction following surgery, often as a result of too aggressive rehabilitation either by the therapist or the patient. This study compared the clinical outcomes of patients after TSA who received formal PT with those treated with a home-based, physician-directed program. We hypothesized that patients with a formal postoperative PT protocol would have significantly better postoperative clinical outcomes compared with patients with no formal PT. Both authors (M.A.F and P.St.P.) independently changed their postoperative rehabilitation program from a formal protocol, carefully supervised and directed by physical therapists, to one that is home-based and directed by the orthopedic surgeon, with no involvement of therapists once the patient is discharged from the hospital. The home-based rehabilitation program advocated in this chapter results from collaboration by the two authors after publication of the aforementioned study.

The study initiating this change in practice included all patients undergoing a primary TSA for a diagnosis of primary osteoarthritis between January 2002 and July 2004 as identified from the senior author's (M.A.F.) database. The indication for surgery was a diagnosis of primary osteoarthritis that was unresponsive to nonoperative management. When adequate preoperative radiographs were available, including a true anteroposterior and axillary lateral, the degree of glenoid erosion was graded according to Rispoli et al.[52]

All surgeries were performed by a single, high-volume shoulder and elbow surgeon with more than 10 years of experience before the start of the study period. A deltopectoral approach and subscapularis tenotomy, as well as a single implant, were used in all cases. Beyond surgeon experience, the only major difference in patient care that we could detect was the change in the postoperative rehabilitation.

Before February 2003, patients were routinely prescribed formal PT postoperatively. After February 2003, the senior author stopped prescribing PT and switched to a home-based, physician-directed rehabilitation program. This allowed a unique opportunity to compare 2 consecutive groups of patients: those having a primary TSA between January 2002 and February 2003, combined with formal postoperative PT (group A); and those having a primary TSA between January 2004 and July 2004 with home-based, physician-directed rehabilitation (group B).

For a patient to be included in the study, preoperative data with respect to the outcome data analyzed must have been available. Of the 50 patients eligible for inclusion in group A, 7 were excluded due to incomplete preoperative data, leaving 43 for inclusion. Of the 44 patients eligible for inclusion in group B, 2 were excluded because they lacked preoperative data and 4 patients were lost to follow-up, leaving 38 for inclusion. All patient data were collected in a prospective manner and reviewed retrospectively for the purpose of this study. Data that were available for analysis and comparison between the 2 groups included patient medical records, radiographs, self-assessed ROM, and patient questionnaires.

Patient questionnaires were provided for all visits and the following information was recorded: (1) Visual analog scale (VAS) for pain, (2) VAS for function, (3) American Shoulder and Elbow Surgeons (ASES) score for pain, (4) ASES score for function, (5) total ASES score, (6) Simple Shoulder Test (SST) score, (7) Short Form-36 version 2 (SF-36v2) score, and (8) patient satisfaction (excellent, good, satisfied, or unsatisfied) with the surgery and patient-assessed ROM.

ROM was determined by the patient self-assessment forms as follows: patients were shown pictures of various arm positions in forward flexion, abduction or internal rotation, and were asked to mark the picture which most closely corresponded to their motion. [56] These answers were converted to degrees for forward flexion and abduction. For internal rotation, the pictures corresponded to the gluteal fold, sacrum, L5, L1, T12, and T6. These, in turn, were given numeric values from 0 (gluteal fold) to 8 (T6) for statistical analysis. Results for internal rotation are reported both by spinal level and numerically.

The postoperative rehabilitation protocols are summarized below with the group A patients receiving formal PT in a 4-phase rehabilitation program supervised by a physical therapist, as follows:

- Phase I (weeks 0 to 3): An immobilizer was used at all times, except during bathing and exercising; active ROM (AROM) of the elbow, wrist and hand; and supine passive ROM (PROM) to a maximum of 20° of external rotation (ER) and 120° of elevation in the scapular plane (scaption).
- Phase II (weeks 4 to 6): Patients continued to use the immobilizer, except during bathing and exercising. Patients progressed to resisted elbow, wrist, and hand exercises; supine active-assisted ROM (AAROM) of the shoulder with a wand, isometric shoulder exercises, and closed chain kinetic shoulder exercises.
- Phase III (weeks 7 to 9): The immobilizer was discontinued. AAROM of the shoulder, isometrics, and closed chain kinetics were continued; and supine and prone AROM of the shoulder was initiated.
- Phase IV: Added were shoulder AROM in the standing position, resistive strengthening exercises, and activities of daily living (ADLs).

The group B patients received a physician-directed rehabilitation program, as follows:

- Phase I: Patients wore immobilizers for 6 to 8 weeks, except during bathing and pendulum exercises.
- Phase II: After 6 to 8 weeks, the patients returned for follow-up, the immobilizer use was discontinued, and they were given a sling to wear when leaving the house. In addition to performing supine, active-assisted forward flexion exercises from this follow-up visit, patients were allowed to use their arms for ADLs.
- Phase III: After 14 weeks, the patients were allowed to participate in any activities they chose that comfort and confidence allowed.

Patient demographic data were compared between groups A and B and no significant differences were detected with regard to age, gender, preoperative ROM, or functional scores (SST and ASES), except for internal rotation, which was significantly better in group A (L1) than group B (L5; P=.02; Table I, Table II). Adequate preoperative radiographs were available for 35 patients from group A and 36 from group B. In group A, 7 patients had no glenoid erosion, 17 had mild, 10 had moderate, and 1 had severe erosion. In group B, 8 patients had no glenoid erosion, 16 had mild, 12 had moderate, and 0 had severe glenoid erosion. There were no significant differences between the 2 groups (Table I). No glenoid bone grafting was required in any patients from either group.

Postoperative data were collected for patients at 3, 6, and 12 months, and at the most recent follow-up. This was at an average of 52 months (range 24-82 months) for group A and 39 months (range 24-51 months) for group B. When preoperative and postoperative data were compared, group A had significant improvements in ASES and SST at all time points evaluated (Table II). Initially, forward flexion and abduction showed significant improvement at 3, 6, and 12 months; however, the improvements in forward flexion preoperatively vs postoperatively (102° vs 119°, P=0.24) and abduction (73°vs 108°, P=.053) did not reach significance at final follow-up (Table II). Internal rotation in group A did not show significant improvement at any time point (Table II).

Group B had significant improvements in ASES, SST, forward flexion, and abduction at all time points (Table II). The physical component summary (PCS) of the SF-36v2 was also significantly improved postoperatively in group B. Compared with preoperative internal rotation, postoperative internal rotation was significantly improved at 6 and 12 months in group B, but this improvement was not sustained at final follow-up (1.6 vs 2.6, P=.053).

When the postoperative values were compared between groups A and B, few differences reached significance (Table II). No differences were detected in the ASES or SST scores at any time point evaluated. A difference was detected in internal rotation at 3 months that was better in group A (L1) than in group B (L5; P=.002). This difference was not sustained, however, and no differences were seen at further follow-up. Conversely, although no differences were detected in forward flexion and abduction between groups at 3, 6, and 12 months, significant differences were seen at final follow-up. Group B showed significantly more forward flexion (154° vs 119°, P=.024) and abduction (147° vs 108°, P=.03) than group A (Table II). Group B also showed a significantly better PCS of 43 compared with group A (43 vs 38, P=.037).

Patient satisfaction was also compared. In group A, 88% of patients were satisfied (excellent, good, and satisfied), with 54% rating their outcome as excellent. Group B reported higher satisfaction, with 95% of patients being satisfied and 76% rating their outcome as excellent. The results of $\chi2$ analysis of satisfied and excellent patients between groups A and B were not significant ($\chi2$ = 0.471; P = .4924; $\chi2$ = 3.162, P = .0754, respectively).

The use of a formal physical therapy program has been accepted as the "gold standard" following shoulder surgery. However, this has not been established to be more effective in obtaining a better clinical outcome than that of a physician supervised home-based physical therapy program. In an effort to study this, the reviewed study was undertaken to determine if the clinical results following formal therapy was significantly better than a home-based program. This study supports the findings of previous studies that TSA has been shown to be a successful procedure for glenohumeral osteoarthritis. It provides significant and lasting improvements in pain relief, function, and patient satisfaction. [17, 43, 45] Improvements were noted in both groups for ROM and functional scores, including ASES, SST, and SF-36 PCS. Interestingly, although group A initially showed significant improvements in forward flexion and abduction, these improvements were not maintained at final follow-up. Significant improvements were maintained at final follow-up in group A for ASES and SST scores. Group B, however, made significant improvements in forward flexion, abduction, ASES, SST, and SF-36 PCS that were maintained at final follow-up. The failure to maintain ROM in group A could be related to the therapy program, the longer follow-up (52 months vs 39 months), or other factors that could not be accounted for in this study. Nevertheless, patients in both groups were very satisfied with their outcomes (88% in group A and 95% in group B).

Although much has been published about outcomes after TSA, little attention has been given to postoperative PT programs or their effects on final outcomes. Boardman et al[7] compared postoperative ROM with preoperative and intraoperative ROM. With a simple, home-based PT program, the postoperative ROM was comparable to the ROM obtained intraoperatively. Most studies in the English literature that have evaluated the results of TSA in patients with primary osteoarthritis, give little or no details regarding the postoperative therapy, and those that are mentioned vary widely from no therapy to intensive, inpatient PT. None of the studies, and no others that we are aware of, directly compare postoperative PT protocols.

Interestingly, the multicenter study by Norris and Iannotti [45] allowed the postoperative PT protocol to be at the treating surgeon's discretion. Nevertheless, the authors state that the outcomes were uniform, although no comparison of outcomes according to the treating surgeon was performed. This study suggests that the postoperative PT protocol may not have a significant effect on the outcome of TSA for primary osteoarthritis. The results show that a simple home therapy program does not negatively affect the outcomes after TSA for primary arthritis. In fact, group B performed better than group A in all parameters and at all time points except internal rotation and abduction at 3 months after TSA.

The strengths of the study include 2 patient populations that appear well matched and a short gap of less than 1 year between the end of the collection period for group A and the start of the collection period for the group B. In addition, all procedures were performed by a single surgeon using the same operative technique and a single implant.

This study has several weaknesses, however. First, the retrospective nature of the study presented problems with our data analysis. Although our data were collected prospectively in the clinic as a routine part of patient follow-up, some of the records did not contain data for every time point evaluated. Therefore, the number of patients in each group varied depending on the information available.

Second, the patients are two consecutive series of patients treated during different time periods. Although, the surgeon made no significant changes in surgical technique and already had more than 10 years of experience, group B was treated later, and the experience gained over time could be considered learner bias.

Third, subtle differences in the patient population or other confounding variables that might influence outcome could not be accounted for.

Fourth, we had no way of measuring patient compliance with the postoperative rehabilitation protocols. This would be particularly important for group A, because outcomes could certainly be influenced by compliance with the PT protocol.

Finally, the average follow-up was different between the 2 groups, and the length of follow-up could influence some of the outcomes measured.

RECOMMENDED PROTOCOL

In an effort to standardize a home-based rehabilitation program for most shoulder surgeries, we have developed a program that includes safe, simple exercises that can be easily reproduced in the home environment. These exercises do not require specialized equipment and can be performed after viewing a web-based program that can be repeatedly viewed by patients at their leisure and based on their need. Just as with all other programs, the initial emphasis is on protection of rotator cuff repair, slow restoration of passive motion to avoid stiffness, progressive active assisted motion, gradual strengthening and return to activities of daily living. By focusing on patient-oriented, home-based therapy programs, we allow patients to take full responsibility for their recovery and not rely on an outside agency to be responsible for their result.

Previous authors have evaluated muscle activity during shoulder rehabilitation exercises and have noted substantial activity even during simple, light exercises. Although this activity is desired for rehabilitation once the rotator cuff has healed, excessive forces are to be avoided while the healing is taking place. This is as true for the repair of the subscapularis following arthroplasty as it is for primary rotator cuff repair. A motivated patient, with the correct guidance, may be the best person to manage their therapy. Pain is a Core strengthening and scapular stabilization are two components of shoulder rehabilitation that are often neglected. Failure to address these components may lead to scapular dyskinesis and asymmetry. [20, 34, 38] These components are easily included in the following protocol using simple to follow exercises that can be performed at home.

Perhaps the most important visit, either with a therapist or with a physician's assistant, would be in the preoperative period. Often termed "prehabilitation", a session or two of instruction to go over the postoperative rehabilitation program is very helpful to the patient. Emphasis is placed on understanding the goals of therapy and practicing their exercises before they experience postoperative pain and immobilization. Immediate postoperative issues such as dressing, bathing, and activities of daily living are addressed so that the patient feels comfortable with those activities prior to surgery. This is very important for elderly patients who live alone and are concerned about their ability to comply with the restrictions following surgery.

- •Phase 0: (prehabilitation)
  All phases of recovery and rehabilitation are reviewed and practiced with patient
  Activities of daily living are practiced in a sling to simulate recovery
- Phase I (weeks 0 to 3):
  Cryotherapy is recommended.
  An immobilizer is to be used at all times, except during bathing and exercising;
  Core strengthening exercises: Single-leg stand against door; lawnmower starts in sling;
  Active ROM (AROM) of the elbow, wrist and hand;
  Scapular/ deltoid exercises: Scapular contractions.
- Phase II (weeks 4 to 6):
  Cryotherapy is recommended following exercises.
  An immobilizer is to be used at all times, except during bathing and exercising;
  Active ROM (AROM) of the elbow, wrist and hand;
  Scapular/ deltoid exercises: Scapular contractions; deltoid isometric exercises in sling;
  Core strengthening exercises: Single-leg stand - unsupported; lawnmower starts in sling;
  Initiate table slides[1] and supported pendulum exercises.
  Initiate AAROM wand exercises in supine position.
- Phase III (weeks 7 to 12):
  The immobilizer is discontinued;
  Scapular/ deltoid exercises: Scapular rows with theraband; deltoid strengthening with theraband;
  Core strengthening exercises: Single-leg stand -unsupported; wall sits and squats;
  Continue table slides and unsupported pendulum exercises as warm-up.

[1] Table slides are accomplished in a seated position by placing the hand of the affected extremity on a table and pushing the arm forward passively by flexion of the body at the waist. Alternative exercises include bowing exercises or desk slides. Desk slides are performed by placing the hand on a desk and sitting on a rolling chair or stool. The passive motion is accomplished by pushing the chair backwards with the legs to generate passive motion of the shoulder. Bowing is accomplished by placing the hand on a higher platform and bowing forward to generate passive motion of the shoulder. All three exercises accomplish the same objective and can be directed individually depending on the patient.

Continue AAROM wand exercises in supine position. Add standing wand behind back.
Initiate wall slide program[2]. Wall slides only to full elevation for most tears. Wall slides with lift-off for small tears.

- Phase IV: (weeks 13 to 26)
  Scapular / deltoid / rotator cuff: Theraband exercises to include rows, three-way deltoid, IR and ER. Increase resistance of bands as toleated. Wall push-ups.
  Core strengthening exercises: Transition to exercise ball – crunches / bridges.
  Continue wall slide program. Progress as tolerated to Wall Slides with lift-off, Wall Slides with lowering, Wall Slides with resisted lowering for eccentric strengthening.
  Return to sport as tolerated when indicated by strength, symptoms and demand of the sport.

Post-operative follow-up with the surgeon is recommended at the end of each phase to assess progress with consideration of transition to formal therapy as each case requires. Referral to formal PT should be considered in patients who are developing greater than expected stiffness or if they demonstrate the inability to follow the home-based program.

A formal PT program is also considered after Phase IV if the patient needs assistance to progress to sports specific activity that requires a higher level of performance. We view this as a very important role for the therapist to help the patient enhance their recovery following initial recovery from these surgeries. Once the patient's rotator cuff repair (as the primary procedure or as part of an arthroplasty) has healed, therapists are extremely effective in evaluating scapular dynamics and can direct therapy to correct any residual dyskinesia. In doing this, the therapist can fine tune shoulder function and focus on return to

---

[2] Wall slide progression starts with pushing the hand up the wall to achieve forward flexion. Initially, the non-operative hand can be used to assist. Wall walking with the fingers tends to initiate deltoid and rotator cuff contraction and we feel a sliding motion leads to a more passive exercise. Once range of motion is achieved wall slides with lift-off is initiated. In this exercise the patient performs a wall slide and then lifts the hand off the wall overhead and holds for 3 – 5 seconds. The hand is placed back on the wall and slides down the wall to the starting position. Wall slides with eccentric lowering adds to the lift –off by turning away from the wall and lowering the hand in the scapular plane with the elbow extended. A final phase of this progression is to add weight. The patient uses a 1 lb. weight or water bottle to push up the wall and then lower eccentrically. This technique adds eccentric exercise which has been used in tendon repair rehabilitation.

desired activities and adjusting for any residual disability following surgery. Such activities may include tennis, golf, weight lifting or yoga.

The results of this review and the TSA study may have significant financial implications. As the burden of health care costs continues to rise, reducing or eliminating spending is becoming more important. A typical 1-hour PT visit is estimated to cost $100. Considering that the number of shoulder surgeries is increasing, the cost of PT after TSA places a significant financial burden on the health care system. Any estimation of cost would also fail to account for the lost time and cost of traveling to the therapy visits, not only for the patients but also for their caregivers who must sacrifice their time to travel with the patient. Increasing, a larger portion of the PT costs are borne by the patient in the form of co-pays in addition to their health insurance premium. If patients are prescribed the usual course of two times a week for up to three months, and pay a $20 co-pay, their individual cost can be close to $500. Therefore, if physical therapy is not an essential component to the patients overall outcome, the overall costs of PT places a significant financial burden on an overextended health care system and the patient.

However, we are not advocating the elimination of formal PT. Indeed, we feel strongly that there is an extremely important role for the physical therapist. Formal PT is used in most patients before surgery is considered, and often is effective in decreasing pain, restoring function, and obviating the need for surgical intervention. PT is also useful in the patients described above who are having problems with their home exercise program and need further assistance. For these patients there is an inherent need to have better communication between the therapist and the surgeon to optimize the patient's result. Additionally, we need better outcome studies evaluation not only the effectiveness of treatment, but also its relative value and cost-effectiveness in this changing medical environment.

Conclusion

After review of the published studies, we do not find support that patients with formal postoperative PT have better postoperative clinical outcomes. In fact, in the study reviewed in detail, the data showed that there was no difference between the postoperative rehabilitation groups, with trends towards better outcomes in patients with no formal rehabilitation. This has broad implications, not only for the way in which surgeons must think about postoperative rehabilitation for TSA but also for all shoulder rehabilitation protocols. We propose in this chapter, and are currently using in our practices, a home-based, patient-centered, postoperative PT program for patients undergoing arthroscopic rotator cuff repair, TSA, and r-TSA. Our findings warrant a more rigorous investigation of the uses of formal physical therapy following shoulder surgery with randomized clinical trials. Naturally, a more cost-effective use of formal physical therapy could lead to a substantial reduction in health care expenditures, which would be a welcome change to the ever-rising burden that healthcare places on the economy.

REFERENCES

[1] A 2008 Shoulder Implant Update. *Orthopedic Network News*. 2008; 19:10–13.

[2] Adams JE, Sperling JW, Schleck CD, Harmsen WS, Cofield RH. Outcomes of shoulder arthroplasty in Olmsted County, Minnesota: a population-based study. *Clin Orthop Relat Res.* 2007; 455:176–182. CrossRef

[3] Amstutz HC, Sew Hoy AL, Clarke IC. UCLA anatomic total shoulder arthroplasty. *Clin Orthop Relat Res*. 1981;7–20.

[4] Amstutz HC, Thomas BJ, Kabo JM, Jinnah RH, Dorey FJ. The Dana total shoulder arthroplasty. *J Bone Joint Surg Am*. 1988; 70:1174–1182. MEDLINE

[5] Barrett WP, Franklin JL, Jackins SE, Wyss CR, Matsen FA. Total shoulder arthroplasty. *J Bone Joint Surg Am*. 1987; 69:865–872. MEDLINE

[6] Bell SN, Gschwend N. Clinical experience with total arthroplasty and hemiarthroplasty of the shoulder using the Neer prosthesis. *Int Orthop.* 1986; 10:217–222. MEDLINE | CrossRef

[7] Boardman ND, Cofield RH, Bengtson KA, Little R, Jones MC, Rowland CM. Rehabilitation after total shoulder arthroplasty. *J Arthroplasty*. 2001; 16:483–486.

[8] Boileau P, Avidor C, Krishnan SG, Walch G, Kempf JF, Mole D. Cemented polyethylene versus uncemented metal-backed glenoid components in total shoulder arthroplasty: a prospective, double-blind, randomized study. *J Shoulder Elbow Surg*. 2002; 11:351–359. Abstract | Full Text | Full-Text PDF (179 KB) | CrossRef

[9] Boileau P, Watkinson DJ, Hatzidakis AM, Balg F. Grammont reverse prosthesis:design, rationale, and biomechanics. *J Shoulder Elbow Surg.* 2005 Jan-Feb;14(1 Suppl S):147S-161S.

[10] Brems JJ. Rehabilitation following total shoulder arthroplasty. *Clin Orthop Relat Res.* 1994;70–85.

[11] Brenner BC, Ferlic DC, Clayton ML, Dennis DA. Survivorship of unconstrained total shoulder arthroplasty. *J Bone Joint Surg Am.* 1989; 71:1289–1296. MEDLINE

[12] Brown DD, Friedman RJ. Postoperative rehabilitation following total shoulder arthroplasty. *Orthop Clin North Am.* 1998;29:535–547. Abstract | Full Text | Full-Text PDF (872 KB) | CrossRef

[13] Bryant D, Litchfield R, Sandow M, Gartsman GM, Guyatt G, Kirkley A. A comparison of pain, strength, range of motion, and functional outcomes after hemiarthroplasty and total shoulder arthroplasty in patients with osteoarthritis of the shoulder. A systematic review and meta-analysis. *J Bone Joint Surg Am.* 2005;87:1947–1956. MEDLINE

[14] Buess E, Steuber KU, Waibl B. Open versus arthroscopic rotator cuff repair: a comparative view of 96 cases. *Arthroscopy.* 2005 May; 21(5):597-604.

[15] Cameron B, Galatz L, Williams GR. Factors affecting the outcome of total shoulder arthroplasty. *Am J Orthop.* 2001;30:613–623. MEDLINE

[16] Clayton ML, Ferlic DC, Jeffers PD. Prosthetic arthroplasties of the shoulder. *Clin Orthop Relat Res.* 1982;184–191.

[17] Cofield RH. Total shoulder arthroplasty with the Neer prosthesis. *J Bone Joint Surg* Am. 1984;66:899–906.

[18] Deshmukh AV, Koris M, Zurakowski D, Thornhill TS. Total shoulder arthroplasty: long-term survivorship, functional outcome, and quality of life. *J Shoulder Elbow Surg.* 2005;14:471–479. Abstract | Full Text | Full-Text PDF (130 KB) | CrossRef

[19] Edwards TB, Kadakia NR, Boulahia A, Kempf JF, Boileau P, Nemoz C, et al. A comparison of hemiarthroplasty and total shoulder arthroplasty in the treatment of primary glenohumeral osteoarthritis: results of a multicenter study. *J Shoulder Elbow Surg.* 2003;12:207–213. Abstract | Full Text | Full-Text PDF (94 KB) | CrossRef

[20] Escamilla RF, Yamashiro K, Paulos L, Andrews JR. Shoulder muscle activity and function in common shoulder rehabilitation exercises. *Sports Med.*2009;39(8):663-85.

[21] Fehringer EV, Kopjar B, Boorman RS, Churchill RS, Smith KL, Matsen FA. Characterizing the functional improvement after total

shoulder arthroplasty for osteoarthritis. *J Bone Joint Surg Am*. 2002; 84:1349–1353.

[22] Fenlin JM, Frieman BG. Indications, technique, and results of total shoulder arthroplasty in osteoarthritis. *Orthop Clin North Am*. 1998; 29:423–434. Full Text | Full-Text PDF (1061 KB) | CrossRef

[23] Fenlin JM, Ramsey ML, Allardyce TJ, Frieman BG. Modular total shoulder replacement. Design rationale, indications, and results. *Clin Orthop Relat Res*. 1994;37–46.

[24] Fenlin JM, Vaccaro A, Andreychik D, Lin S. Modular total shoulder: early experience and impressions. *Semin Arthroplasty*. 1990;1:102–111. MEDLINE

[25] Frich LH, Moller BN, Sneppen O. Shoulder arthroplasty with the Neer Mark-II prosthesis. Arch Orthop Trauma Surg. 1988;107:110–113. MEDLINE | CrossRef

[26] Gartsman GM, Roddey TS, Hammerman SM. Shoulder arthroplasty with or without resurfacing of the glenoid in patients who have osteoarthritis. J Bone Joint Surg Am. 2000;82:26–34. MEDLINE

[27] Gartsman GM, Russell JA, Gaenslen E. Modular shoulder arthroplasty. J Shoulder Elbow Surg. 1997;6:333–339. MEDLINE | CrossRef

[28] Gerber C, Pennington SD, Nyffeler RW. Reverse total shoulder arthroplasty. *J Am Acad Orthop Surg*. 2009 May;17(5):284-95.

[29] Godeneche A, Boileau P, Favard L, Le Huec JC, Levigne C, Nove-Josserand L, et al. Prosthetic replacement in the treatment of osteoarthritis of the shoulder: early results of 268 cases. *J Shoulder Elbow Surg*. 2002; 11:11–18. Abstract | Full Text | Full-Text PDF (220 KB) | CrossRef

[30] Godeneche A, Boulahia A, Noel E, Boileau P, Walch G. Total shoulder arthroplasty in chronic inflammatory and degenerative disease. *Rev Rhum Engl Ed*. 1999;66:560–570. MEDLINE

[31] Goldberg BA, Smith K, Jackins S, Campbell B, Matsen FA. The magnitude and durability of functional improvement after total shoulder arthroplasty for degenerative joint disease. *J Shoulder Elbow Surg*. 2001;10:464–469. Abstract | Full Text | Full-Text PDF (220 KB) | CrossRef

[32] Gristina AG, Romano RL, Kammire GC, Webb LX. Total shoulder replacement. *Orthop Clin North Am*. 1987;18:445–453. MEDLINE

[33] Hawkins RJ, Bell RH, Jallay B. Total shoulder arthroplasty. *Clin Orthop Relat Res*. 1989;188–194.

[34] Huberty DP, Schoolfield JD, Brady PC, Vadala AP, Arrigoni P, Burkhart SS. Incidence and treatment of postoperative stiffness following arthroscopic rotator cuff repair. *Arthroscopy*. 2009 Aug; 25(8):880-90.

[35] Hughes M, Neer CS. Glenohumeral joint replacement and postoperative rehabilitation. *Phys Ther*. 1975;55:850–858. MEDLINE

[36] Iannotti JP, Norris TR. Influence of preoperative factors on outcome of shoulder arthroplasty for glenohumeral osteoarthritis. *J Bone Joint Surg Am*. 2003;85:251–258.

[37] Jackins S. Postoperative shoulder rehabilitation. *Phys Med Rehabil Clin N Am*. 2004;15(vi):643–682. Full Text | Full-Text PDF (686 KB) | CrossRef

[38] Koo SS, Burkhart SS. Rehabilitation following arthroscopic rotator cuff repair. *Clin Sports Med*. 2010 Apr;29(2):203-11

[39] Lo IK, Litchfield RB, Griffin S, Faber K, Patterson SD, Kirkley A. Quality-of-life outcome following hemiarthroplasty or total shoulder arthroplasty in patients with osteoarthritis. A prospective, randomized trial. *J Bone Joint Surg Am*. 2005;87:2178–2185. MEDLINE

[40] Martin SD, Zurakowski D, Thornhill TS. Uncemented glenoid component in total shoulder arthroplasty. Survivorship and outcomes. *J Bone Joint Surg Am*. 2005; 87:1284–1292. MEDLINE

[41] Mileti J, Sperling JW, Cofield RH, Harrington JR, Hoskin TL. Monoblock and modular total shoulder arthroplasty for osteoarthritis. *J Bone Joint Surg Br*. 2005; 87:496–500.

[42] Millar NL, Wu X, Tantau R, Silverstone E, Murrell GA. Open versus two forms of arthroscopic rotator cuff repair. *Clin Orthop Relat Res*. 2009 Apr; 467(4):966-78.

[43] Neer CS, Watson KC, Stanton FJ. Recent experience in total shoulder replacement. *J Bone Joint Surg Am*. 1982; 64:319–337. MEDLINE

[44] Norris BL, Lachiewicz PF. Modern cement technique and the survivorship of total shoulder arthroplasty. *Clin Orthop Relat Res*. 1996; 76–85.

[45] Norris TR, Iannotti JP. Functional outcome after shoulder arthroplasty for primary osteoarthritis: a multicenter study. J Shoulder Elbow Surg. 2002; 11:130–135. Abstract | Full Text | Full-Text PDF (154 KB) | CrossRef

[46] Orfaly RM, Rockwood CA, Esenyel CZ, Wirth MA. A prospective functional outcome study of shoulder arthroplasty for osteoarthritis with

an intact rotator cuff. *J Shoulder Elbow Surg*. 2003; 12:214–221. Abstract | Full Text | Full-Text PDF (258 KB) | CrossRef

[47] Parsons IM, Campbell B, Titelman RM, Smith KL, Matsen FA. Characterizing the effect of diagnosis on presenting deficits and outcomes after total shoulder arthroplasty. *J Shoulder Elbow Surg*. 2005; 14:575–584. Abstract | Full Text | Full-Text PDF (814 KB) | CrossRef

[48] Pfahler M, Jena F, Neyton L, Sirveaux F, Mole D. Hemiarthroplasty versus total shoulder prosthesis: results of cemented glenoid components. *J Shoulder Elbow Surg*. 2006;15:154–163. Abstract | Full Text | Full-Text PDF (205 KB) | CrossRef

[49] Radnay CS, Setter KJ, Chambers L, Levine WN, Bigliani LU, Ahmad CS. Total shoulder replacement compared with humeral head replacement for the treatment of primary glenohumeral osteoarthritis: a systematic review. *J Shoulder Elbow Surg*. 2007;16:396–402. Abstract | Full Text | Full-Text PDF (99 KB)

[50] Raiss P, Aldinger PR, Kasten P, Rickert M, Loew M. Total shoulder replacement in young and middle-aged patients with glenohumeral osteoarthritis. *J Bone Joint Surg Br*. 2008;90:764–769. CrossRef

[51] Ranawat CS, Warren R, Inglis AE. Total shoulder replacement arthroplasty. *Orthop Clin North Am*. 1980;11:367–373. MEDLINE

[52] Rispoli DM, Sperling JW, Athwal GS, Schleck CD, Cofield RH. Humeral head replacement for the treatment of osteoarthritis. *J Bone Joint Surg Am*. 2006; 88:2637–2644. MEDLINE | CrossRef

[53] Roper BA, Paterson JM, Day WH. The Roper-Day total shoulder replacement. *J Bone Joint Surg Br*. 1990;72:694–697.

[54] Sauerbrey AM, Getz CL, Piancastelli M, Iannotti JP, Ramsey ML, Williams GR Jr. Arthroscopic versus mini-open rotator cuff repair: a comparison of clinical outcome. *Arthroscopy*. 2005 Dec;21(12):1415-20.

[55] Severud EL, Ruotolo C, Abbott DD, Nottage WM. All-arthroscopic versus mini-open rotator cuff repair: A long-term retrospective outcome comparison. *Arthroscopy*. 2003 Mar;19(3):234-8.

[56] Smith AM, Barnes SA, Sperling JW, Farrell CM, Cummings JD, Cofield RH. Patient and physician-assessed shoulder function after arthroplasty. *J Bone Joint Surg Am*. 2006;88:508–513. MEDLINE

[57] Sperling JW, Cofield RH, Rowland CM. Minimum fifteen-year follow-up of Neer hemiarthroplasty and total shoulder arthroplasty in patients aged fifty years or younger. *J Shoulder Elbow Surg*. 2004;13:604–613. Abstract | Full Text | Full-Text PDF (264 KB) | CrossRef

[58] Sperling JW, Cofield RH, Rowland CM. Neer hemiarthroplasty and Neer total shoulder arthroplasty in patients fifty years old or less. Long-term results. *J Bone Joint Surg Am.* 1998;80:464–473. MEDLINE

[59] Taunton MJ, McIntosh AL, Sperling JW, Cofield RH. Total shoulder arthroplasty with a metal-backed, bone-ingrowth glenoid component. Medium to long-term results. *J Bone Joint Surg Am.* 2008;90:2180–2188. CrossRef

[60] Torchia ME, Cofield RH, Settergren CR. Total shoulder arthroplasty with the Neer prosthesis: long-term results. *J Shoulder Elbow Surg.* 1997;6:495–505. MEDLINE | CrossRef

[61] van de Sande MA, Brand R, Rozing PM. Indications, complications, and results of shoulder arthroplasty. *Scand J Rheumatol.* 2006;35:426–434. MEDLINE | CrossRef

[62] van de Sande MA, Rozing PM. Modular total shoulder system with short stem. A prospective clinical and radiological analysis. *Int Orthop.* 2004;28:115–118. MEDLINE | CrossRef

[63] Wallace AL, Phillips RL, MacDougal GA, Walsh WR, Sonnabend DH. Resurfacing of the glenoid in total shoulder arthroplasty. A comparison, at a mean of five years, of prostheses inserted with and without cement. *J Bone Joint Surg Am.* 1999;81:510–518. MEDLINE

[64] Weiss AP, Adams MA, Moore JR, Weiland AJ. Unconstrained shoulder arthroplasty. A five-year average follow-up study. *Clin Orthop Relat Res.* 1990;86–90.

[65] Wilcox RB, Arslanian LE, Millett P. Rehabilitation following total shoulder arthroplasty. *J Orthop Sports Phys Ther.* 2005;35:821–836. MEDLINE

In: Physical Therapy
Editor: James P. Bennett
ISBN: 978-1-61122-418-4

Chapter 5

ISOKINETIC ASSESSMENT AND MUSCLE STRENGTH TRAINING USED IN PEOPLE WITH MULTIPLE SCLEROSIS

Jean-François Aubry, Emmanuel Rose, Karine Petrel, Benoit Nicolas, Sandrine Robineau and Philippe Gallien *

Center of Physical Medecine and Rehabilitation
of Saint Helier, Rennes, France

ABSTRACT

Muscle weakness is a main factor of neurological impairment in several diseases such as multiple sclerosis, cerebral palsy and stroke patients. Several studies have stressed that, in such a situation, muscle strength training results in functional improvement. Reliable and reproducible, isokinetic evaluation can quantify a motor deficit and guide the muscle groups through strength training. When the quadriceps suffer a level of decifiect, which causes one to reduce the speed at which they walk, as aresult the hamstring muscles will weaken causing a greater disability. Isokinetic strengthening of the muscle groups with no consequence on spasticity, provides significant functional results. In

* Correspondance : Dr P Gallien, Center of Physical Medecine and Rehabilitation of Saint Helier, 54, rue Saint Hélier , 35 000 Rennes, France, e-mail: philippe.gallien@polempr-sthelier.com

multiple sclerosis, regular muscule strengthening allows the patient to maintain or even improve functional levels, making isokinetic strengthening relevant. After an isokinetic evaluation, the patient's deficits are taken into consideration and a protocol of rehabilitation, which usually includes strength training, is defined. Three protocols are identified. The first one involves the recurvatum of the knee, the second involves strengthening the quad-riceps and the third focuses on hip flexors. This type of isokinetic training, which is associated with a standard multidisciplinary approach, possesses an important functional interest including: transfer, climb and descent of staircases, and improving gait (speed, quality and endurance). However, due to the evolution of the disease, regular follow-up visits are important and necessary.

Multiple sclerosis (MS) is an inflammatory disease of the central nervous system, which affects young people and mostly adult women. The consecutive handicap varies in patients, depending on the localization and the course of the disease: relapsing, remitting or progressive. Motor disorders are frequent with muscle weakness, balance troubles and spasticity [1,2].

People suffering from MS often limit their level of physical activity in order to avoid risking exacerbation, a symptom of this chronic illness. However, decreasing physical activity tends to increase deconditioning, which as a result, alters one's level of fitness [3,4,5].Thus, we must ask ourselves: is muscle strengthening beneficial for people with MS?

The muscle weakness experienced by those suffering from MS stems from a reduced maximum voluntary contraction force, which alters the central motor drive. Isokinetic assessment shows this deficit even in patients with low EDSS. [6,7, 8,9]. This deficit may play a role in the attenuated response to maximal exercise testing. Atrophy exceeding that, which was observed in short-term disuse and approaching that, which was reported in spinal cord injury was observed in MS patients. Muscles presented fewer type I fibers and fibers of all types were smaller with reduced enzyme activities, consistent with results observed in models of disuse [4,8].

Isokinetic tools have been used to assess muscle weakness in central neurological disorders. They are reproducible as well as sensitive. A correlation has been demonstrated between muscle weaknesses and walking parameters, thus the speed at which one comfortably walks is linked to hamstring strength. Quadricep strength could also have an influence on quick walking speed in patients with sensitive disorders or a high level of impairment.

Isokinetic assessment was used in the evaluation of gait disorders. Links were observed between muscle weakness and gait disorders in multiple sclerosis and stroke patients. This supports the hypothesis that muscle strengthening can improve gait impairment. [9,10,11,12,13,14]

Muscular weakness assessment in central neurology can be done at two levels. The first step is the analytic assessment followed by the functional analysis, which is the second step and focuses on the realization and selectivity of movement. In the last 20 years, several authors have demonstrated the possibility of using isokinetic tests in the evaluation of muscular deficit in MS [6,7,9,14] and stroke patients[13,15,16].

Concentric isokinetic tests are reproducible for hip, knee and ankle flexors and extensors especially for low speed. In a previous work, we found a good reproducibility in MS at slow speed (60°/sec) for knee flexors and extensors [6]. Good participation from the patient is needed to obtain reliable results. On the other hand, isokinetic assessment of muscular fatigue does not have a good reproducibility.

A lack of sensitivity in usual muscular testing, notably in the case of moderate deficit, has been demonstrated. Muscular testing does not reflect the degree of muscular deficit dynamically and, after rehabilitation, it is not sensitive enough to evaluate the increase in maximum strength. This has already been stressed by Davies [17] and Watkins [15]. Sunnerhagen compared hemiplegic patients with a matched group and was able to show that a motor deficit was not found during testing of the so-called "healthy" side [18]. This could be linked to their extremely sedentary lifestyle, an effect of the handicap, and a modification of the muscle fibers.

Muscular spasticity does not seem to be a problem when lower than three on the Aschworth scale. In his study on hemiplegic patients, Sharp [13] did not report a relation between the relaxation index in the pendulum test and peak strength. However, a decrease in maximum peak strength of extremely spastic hemiplegic patients (Aschworth > 3) was reported.

Several isokinetic protocols have been proposed: number and type of session, number and modalities of muscle contractions (eccentric or concentric), and contraction speeds vary according to the different published studies. In most of the cases training programs last six weeks, with three sessions per week and are associated with conventional rehabilitation. A period of warm-up precedes isokinetic strengthening. The number of series varies from three to 15 with the number of repetitions between six and ten. The used speeds are between 30°/sec and 180°/sec in concentric, and between 15°/sec and 180°/sec in eccentric. The peak torque at 30°/sec is correlated to the peak torque at a higher speed.

A good contraction of the agonist muscle is obtained with the eccentric mode without reflex contraction of the antagonist muscle, which is often seen in central neurological disorders. Moreover, eccentric strengthening improves both eccentric and concentric strength, and has no influence on muscle spasticity. It also increases fitness and has a positive impact on fatigue sensation. Results on functional status also depend on physical disability such as stance disorders. A correlation between gait disorders and specific muscle deficits have been reported. Thus it justifies strengthening specific muscles with isokinetics. Functional improvement can be maintained over a course of three months, which means that the patients must have regular medical follow ups. In order to improve functional results, resistance training can be used in correlation with endurance training.

We have developed different protocols according to the clinical status of patients during inpatient or outpatient rehabilitation programs.

At the onset, a concentric isokinetic assessment is always performed. Peak torque of extensors and flexors are recorded using a contrex isokinetic dynamometer with five repetitions at 60°/sec and 180°/sec. Then, using the results of this evaluation along with the clinical data (walking, stair climbing abilities, etc.) a specific program of strength training is proposed either for the knee, hip or sometimes for both joints.

Knee protocol for recurvatum consists in seven series of eight repetitions of eccentric contractions at a speed of 15°/sec, with a rest period of one minute between each series, using a visual feedback.

The target of the second protocol is eccentric quadricep strengthening in the case of a knee extensor deficit with failure to stand at the same speed. In this particular case the EDSS score is often higher than in the previous situation.

The third protocol concerns a hip flexor deficit with sessions of five series of five eccentric repetitions.

Now, we will report our findings from a study in which we observed particular patients undergoing rehabilitation for walking problems, and in whom we found a unilateral recurvatum of the knee. The aims of the study were to quantify the suspected muscular deficit in view of the recurvatum, to trea the recurvatum of the knee by eccentric strengthening of the hamstrings, as well as long-term functional and muscular evaluation during rehabilitation.

Inclusion criteria were:

- Patients suffering from MS (diagnosis verified by the MS clinic neurologists)
- Presence of a unilateral recurvatum when walking

- Inferior spasticity of three on the modified Aschworth scale (8)
- Feasible isokinetic test

The initial assessment consisted of a clinical examination with manual muscular testing, evaluation of spasticity on the modified Aschworth scale as well as a concentric isokinetic test on the Cybex Norm. Furthermore, the patients quantified their degree of satisfaction with their gait on a Visual Analogue Scale.

The same protocol was applied at the end of the period of rehabilitation, and at three months. The rehabilitation protocol of 12 sessions was carried out in our rehabilitation center. Each session consisted of eccentric isokinetic muscle strengthening of the hamstrings at slow speed (from 15 to 25°/sec) with visual biofeedback: 50 repetitions at each session in series of seven with a rest of two minutes between each series. This strengthening was combined with a neuro-motor rehabilitation of the gait: learning to control the knee and working on the gait.

On completion of treatment, advice on maintaining regular physical activity was given.

28 voluntary patients (19 women, 9 men) with an average age of 46.6 years +/- 7.2 (34-62) presenting with, most frequently, a progressive form (25 cases) and capable of walking (average EDSS: 4+/-0.7 (3-6) (figure n° 1).

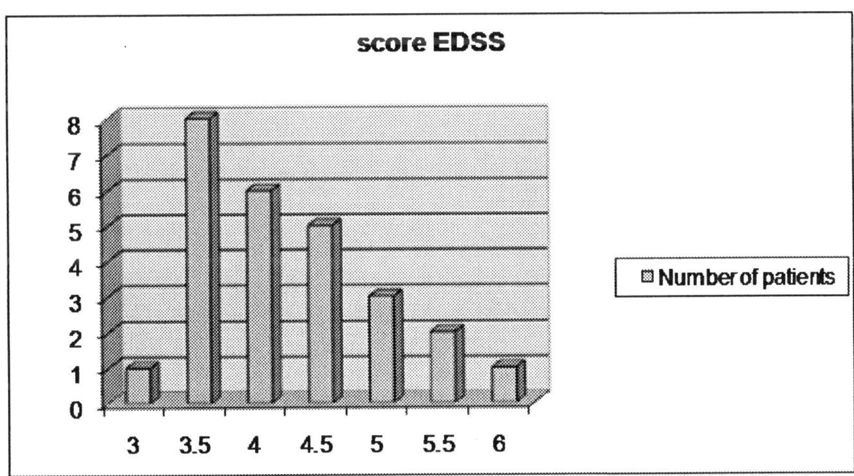

Figure 1. EDSS score of the population.

In 19 cases the recurvatum was on the right, in nine on the left. The associated neurological symptoms were cerebellar in seven cases, and proprioceptive in 16 cases. The evaluation of muscular spasticity on the modified Aschworth scale found an average value of 1.1 +/-1 (0-3).

The initial manual testing evaluated the quadriceps on the deficient side at 4 +/-0.7 (3-5) and the hamstrings at 3.2 +/-0.5 (2-4).

For statistical analysis we have used the non-parametric Wilcoxon test.

At the end of the study the following results were noticed.

Auto-evaluation by VAS showed an average initial score of 3.6 +/-1.5 (0-7). At the end of rehabilitation it had risen to 6.5 +/-1.5 (3-9) . The recurvatum had been improved in 26 cases or had disappeared at slow walking speed (1.5 km/h). In seven cases we remarked reappearance at fast speed (2.5 km/h) on a treadmill. In two patients the recurvatum had not disappeared.

The final manual testing carried out by the same examiner showed no change. No aggravation of spasticity was noted (comparable Aschworth score). There was no neurological aggravation during the sessions.

One incident took place: appearance of pain in the hamstrings requiring a break of one week with no further problems when rehabilitation was restarted.

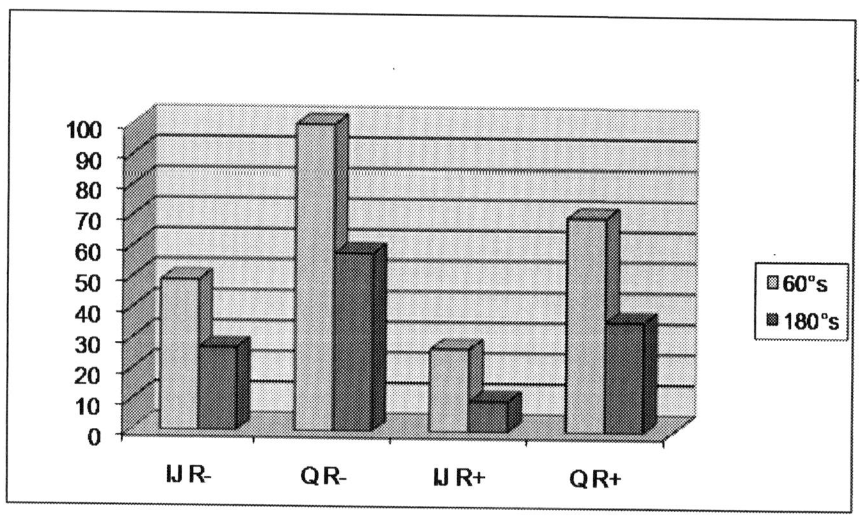

Figure 2. Peak torque of quadriceps and hamstring before rehabilitation R+ : side of recurvatum, R- : side without recurvatum.

On the first isokinetic assessment, there was a significant deficit in the hamstrings on the side with recurvatum (R+) but also in the quadriceps at the two speeds (figure 2). The peak torque of the hamstrings had a value of 26,9 +/-21 on the affected side for a value of 48.9 +/- 16,8 on the unaffected side at a speed of 60°/sec, at the speed of at180°/sec the values were respectively of 10.4 +/-10.6 and 27.1 +/- 11.4. For the quadriceps the registered values were: 70.2 +/- 34.6 at 60°/sec and 36.4 +/- 15.29 at 180°/sec on the affected side versus 99.9 +/- 33.8 and 58 .1 +/- 19.5 (figure 3).

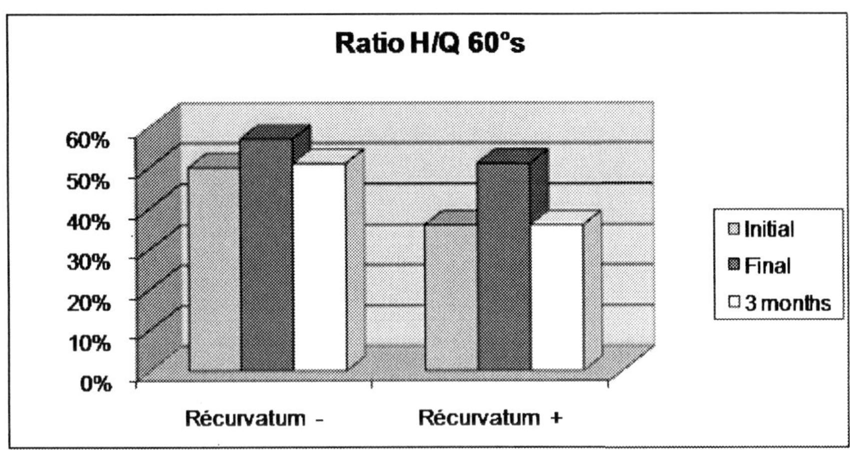

Figure 3. Outcome of the ratio of the hamstrings to the quadriceps before and after rehabilitation at 60 °/sec.

On both sides, in the hamstrings and in the quadriceps, the increase of muscle strength was statistically significant after rehabilitation (p<0.001). (Table 1)

Table 1: Isokinetic Assessment and outcome of the peak torque of the hamstrings and the quadriceps at the speeds of 60 °/sec and 180 °/sec

	Initial		End of rehabilitation		3 months	
	affected	unaffected	affected	unaffected	affected	unaffected
Hamstrings 60°/sec	48.9 +/- 16.8	26.9 +/- 21.4	57.9 +/- 18	41.4 +/- 20.1	50.3 +/- 16.3	26.8 +/- 18.6
Quadriceps 60°/sec	99.9 +/- 33.8	70 .2 +/- 34.6	102.8 +/- 29.1	80.4 +/- 32.2	100.05 +/- 24.2	73.4 +/- 28.6
Hamstrings 180°/sec	27.1 +/- 11.4	10.4 +/- 10.6	35 2 +/- 12.7	20.6 +/- 12.5	29.2 +/- 11.5	13 +/- 11
Quadriceps 180°/sec	58 .11 +/- 19.5	36.4 +/- 15.3	60.5 +/- 17.7	42.14 +/- 18.6	56.4 +/- 17.3	39.2 +/- 14.9

Figure 3 and 4 show the development of the ratio of the hamstrings to the quadriceps before and after rehabilitation. Before rehabilitation this ratio had plummeted on the side with recurvatum (36% at 60°/sec and 28% at180°/sec) at the two speeds. It neared normal after rehabilitation and became comparable to the so-called healthy side).

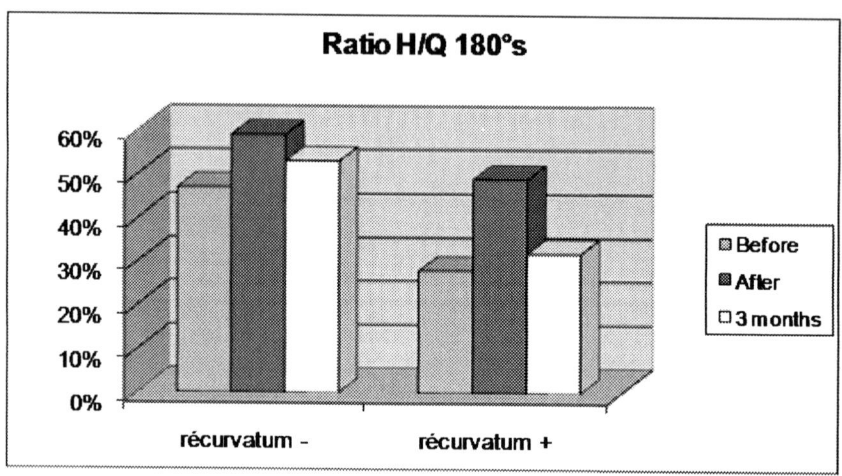

Figure 4. Outcome of the ratio of the hamstrings to the quadriceps before and after rehabilitation at 180 °/sec.

On average at three months a return to the previous state was noted, whether it be the absolute value or in the ratio HS/Q (table 1, and figure 4 and 5). On the other hand, the score for assessment of the quality of walking remained at the same level (VAS = 6.2 +/-1 (4-8)).

DISCUSSION

The clinical condition of MS varies from day to day, this being a characteristic of the disease even in the absence of a flare-up. A feeling of fatigue can frequently interfere.

Therefore we chose to use isokinetic tools, which also provide the advantage of being a dynamic method of evaluation more closely linked to the physiology. Moreover the rehabilitation was carried out in eccentric mode, which did not increase the contraction of antagonists.

The results confirm the possibility of increasing the maximum muscle strength in MS as it has been published for other neurological pathologies [19, 20, 21, 22] . Similar to Sharp [13], the results for absolute value of peak strength do not hold up in the long-term, but in our case the VAS remains steady and in its case the scale for quality of life remains at a better level, as does the speed of walking.

The problem of the existence of recurvatum in patients with cerebral lesions has already been raised [15] and the involvement of the quadriceps alone has been called into question. A greater deficit in the HS than in the Q was noticed in hemiplegic patients [13, 23]. In our patients, the ratio was inverse on the affected side. The hamstrings play a stabilizing, braking role when changing pace. It would seem logical that their weakness is implicated in the appearance of recurvatum of the knee. Even if it is not possible to attribute the improvement in control of the recurvatum solely to eccentric isokinetic muscle strengthening insofar as the patients also work on neuromuscular co-ordination, this eccentric reinforcement without any increase in spasticity definitely allows a threshold limit of strength to be passed, below which control is impossible. This opens the door to work on actual eccentric muscle strengthening in MS. The observed limits in voluntary control of the recurvatum are the speed of rapid movement, which can make it reappear, and fatigue, according to the day or above a certain distance. This leads to questions being posed about the evaluation criteria of the quality of the gait in the course of monitoring these patients, who can control their knee if asked to do so in the consulting room, but who may report a reappearance of the recurvatum in other circumstances. This may possibly lead to the examiner being more positive than it is the case in everyday life: hence the relevance of auto-evaluation by the patient. The walking speed, given in some publications, for hemiplegics does not necessarily reflect directly on the quality of the gait.

This work underlines the interest of muscle strengthening in MS patients with a major muscle weakness of the hamstrings presenting with recurvatum of the knee. Manual muscular testing had in fact played down this deficit, and therefore we stress its limitations. Our patients have been able to benefit from a short program of eccentric isokinetic muscle strengthening of the hamstrings without any noteworthy incident, without increase in spasticity and with rapid functional improvement.

CONCLUSION

Isokinetic is a useful tool for the assessment of muscle strength in patients suffering from multiple sclerosis, but also for rehabilitation. Muscle strengthening can be proposed in rehabilitation programs with good analytic and functional results.

REFERENCES

[1] Gallien P, Robineau S. Sensory-motor and genito-sphincter dysfunctions in multiple sclerosis. *Biomed Pharmac* 1999, 53: 380-85

[2] Coustant M. Sclérose en plaques : aspects cliniques et diagnostiques. *Neuro-psy 2000* ; 15 (4) : 178-182

[3] Gallien P, Nicolas B, Robineau S, Pétrilli S, Houedakor J, Durufle A. Physical training and multiple sclerosis. *Ann Read Med Phys* 2007 ; 50, 6 : 373-6

[4] Kent-Braun J.A., Sharma K.R., Miller R.G., Weiner M.W. Postexercice phosphocreatine resynthesis is slowed in multiple sclerosis. *Muscle Nerve* 1994; 17: 835-841

[5] Petajan j, White A : Recommendations for physical activity in patients with multiple sclerosis. *Sports Med* 1999 ; 27 (3) :179-191

[6] Armstrong L ; Winant D ; Swasey P ; seidle M ; Carter A ; Gehlsen G : Using isokinetic dynamometry to test ambulatory patients with multiple sclerosis. *Phys Ther* 1983 ; 63, 8: 1274-1279

[7] Joubrel ; B. Nicolas ; S. Robineau ; AC. De Crouy, G. Edan ; R. Brissot ; P. Gallien: Evaluation isocinétique de la flexion extension du genou chez les patients ambulatoires atteints de SEP. *Ann Read Med Phys* 2000 ; 43 : 138-144

[8] Kent-Braun J.A., Castro M, Weiner M.W, Gelinas D, Dudley GA, Miller RG. Strength, skeletal muscle composition and enzyme activity in multiple sclerosis. *J Appl Physiol* 1997; 83:1998-2004

[9] Robineau S, Nicolas B, Gallien P, Petrilli S, Durufle A, Edan G et al. Renforcement musculaire isocinétique excentrique dans la rééducation du recurvatum de genou chez des patients atteints de sclérose en plaque : Résultats préliminaires à 3 mois. *Ann Read Med Phys* 2005 ; 48 :29-33

[10] Cantalloube s, monteil i, lamotte d, mailhan l, thoumie P. Evaluation préliminaire des effets de la rééducation sur les paramètres de force,

d'équilibre et de marche dans la sclérose en plaque. *Ann Read Med Phys* 2006 ; 49 : 143-146

[11] Ponichtera Ja, Rodgers Mm, Glaser Rm, Mathews Ta, Camaione Dn. Concentric and eccentric isokinetic lower extremity strength in multiple sclerosis. *J Orthop Sport Phys Ther* 1992 ; 16 : 114-22

[12] Thoumie P, Lamotte D, Cantalloube S, Faucher M, Amarenco G. Motor determinants of gait in 100 ambulatory patients with multiple sclerosis. *Mult Scler* 2005 ; 11 : 485-491.

[13] Sharp S ; Brouwer B :Isokinetic strength training of hemiparetic knee : effects on function and spasticity. *Arch Phys Med Rehabil* 1997 ; 78 : 1231-1236

[14] Kim C.M., Eng J.J., The relationship of lower-extremity muscle torque to locomotor performance in people with stroke. *Phys Ther*.2003; 83: 49-57.

[15] Watkins MP ; Harris BA ; Kozlowxki BA ; Isokinetic testing in patients with hemiparesis. A pilot study. *Phys Ther* 1984 ; 64 :184-189

[16] Tripp E., Harris S. Test-retest reability of isokinetic knee extension and flexion torque measurements in persons with spastic hemiparesis, *Phys Ther* 1991; 71: 45-51.

[17] Davies JM ; Mayston MJ ; Newham DJ ; : Electrical and mechanical output of the knee muscles during isometric and isokinetic activity in stroke an healthy adults. *Disabil Rehabil* 1996 ; 18 : 83-90

[18] Sunnerhagen K ; Svantesson U ; Lönn L ; Krotkiewski M ; Grimby G : Upper motor neuron lesions : their effect on muscle performance and appearance in stroke patients with minor motor impairment. *Arch Phys Med Rehabil* 1999 ;80 : 155-161

[19] Rouleaud S, Gaujard E, Petit H, Picard D,Dehail P, Joseph PA ; Mazaux JM ; Barat M : Isocinetisme et rééducation de la marche . *Ann Med Phys Read* 2000 ;43 : 428-436

[20] Bjarnadottir OH, Konradsdottir AD, Reynisdottir K, Olafson E. Multiple sclerosis and brief moderate exercise. A randomised study. *Mult Scler* 2007; 13:176-82

[21] Petajan J.H., Gappmaier E., White A.T., Spencer M.K., Mino L., Hicks R. Impact of aerobic training on fitness and quality of life in multiple sclerosis. *Ann. Neurol.* 1996; 39: 432-41

[22] Gutierrez GM, Chow JW, Tillman MD, Mc Coy SC, Castellano V, White LJ. Resistance training improves gait kinematics in persons with multiple sclerosis. *Arch Phys Med Rehabil* 2005; 8-: 1824-9

[23] Engardt M ; Knutsson e ; Jonsson M ; Sternhag M ; : Dynamic muscle strength training in stroke patients : effects on knee extension torque, electromyographic activity and motor function. *Arch Phys Med Rehabil* 1995 ;76 : 419-425

In: Physical Therapy
Editor: James P. Bennett
ISBN: 978-1-61122-418-4

Chapter 6

TRADITIONAL MIRROR THERAPY (TMT) IN THE PHYSICAL THERAPY MANAGEMENT OF MOVEMENT AND POSTURAL CONTROL PROBLEMS *

Martin J. Watson
School of Allied Health Professions (AHP) & Health and Social Sciences Research Institute, Faculty of Health, University of East Anglia (UEA), Norwich, UK

INTRODUCTION

Mirrors have a long history as an 'essential' piece of rehabilitation equipment, and can be found in many physical therapy treatment areas. Traditionally one of their main uses is to provide patients with a reflected body image of themselves, usually as (a component of) a therapeutic strategy aimed at retraining movement control and posture. For example, when as a result of central nervous system (CNS) damage such as stroke, people have impaired postural control, then therapists might provide them within a reflected mirror

*A verison of this chapter was also published in *Handbook of Motor Skills: Develpoment, Impairment and Therapy,* edited by Lucian T. Pelligrino, published by Nova Science Publishers, Inc. It was submitted for appropriate modifications in an effort to encourage wider dissemination of research.

image of themselves to deliver augmented visual feedback during treatment sessions where motor training is occurring.

There has recently been much interest in the therapeutic use of mirrors placed perpendicular to the patient's coronal plane; i.e mirrors able to reflect an image of one limb onto the limb of the opposite body side. Recent works by researchers such as Ramachandran [1-4], and Sutbeyaz and Yavuzer [5, 6], have indicated that this may be a useful therapeutic strategy in instances where CNS pathology has resulted in unilateral instances of paresis, neglect or phantom pain. So for example, a mirror might be used to reflect the left (sound) arm onto the right (paralysed) arm following a stroke, as part of a therapeutic strategy aiming to rehabilitate movement on the affected side. One proposed mechanism is that reflection creates an illusion of normal movement/sensation on the affected side of the body, thus facilitating voluntary production of movement and/or normal sensory processing on that side.

Whilst this newer work, now often referred to as 'mirror therapy', is advancing, the original more traditional and (possibly) simpler therapeutic use of mirrors described at the start appears to be being somewhat overlooked and neglected. In this more traditional context (hereafter referred to as 'Traditional Mirror Therapy' or TMT), a full length body mirror is typically placed in front of the person (i.e. parallel to their coronal plane), thus providing them with a full frontal image of their body and its movements. In this way the person is provided with augmented (visual) feedback of their postural alignment and/or bodily movement. This might typically be carried out in conjunction with corrective instructions from the therapist.

One of the puzzles regarding TMT is the apparent absence of any evidence base or instructional advice for what is in effect a fairly simple and straightforward training strategy with a seemingly long history. The notion of therapist/educator-provided augmented feedback during (motor) learning is a well established one; in a recent narrative review for example, van Vliet and Wulf identified a reasonably substantial (albeit nascent) evidence base for this general strategy for motor skills training following stroke [7]. They identified verbal, visual, video and kinematic feedback strategies as the main ones which have been used and evaluated by therapists working with this very common patient group. Interestingly however, this overview did not identify any literature relating to TMT. Similarly, if one accesses key physical therapy instructional texts, there is usually a very limited amount of information on TMT. For example, in a fairly seminal UK text, Howe and Oldham [8] state that "*Full length mirrors are frequently used in physiotherapy departments to make patients more aware of their static posture either in sitting or standing and dynamic posture during movement. Mirrors are also employed in gait retraining...*" (p.237). Howevere no further details are provided.

It is perhaps not difficult to explain this dearth of information regarding TMT. Despite its longstanding presence in the physical therapist's armamentarium, it is easily conceivable that the approach has yet to receive the level of investigation and exploration which it deserves. The physical therapy evidence base is still in its relative infancy and the majority of existing therapeutic strategies probably await appropriate formal evaluation; TMT is probably no exception in this respect.

The aim of this chapter is to provide an overview of several aspects of TMT. Specifically, the chapter covers 3 topics, these being:

- Literature: what is known about TMT from published peer-reviewed reports of formal investigations of this strategy
- Recent research: an overview of 3 pilot projects conducted by the author and colleagues which each evaluate an aspect of TMT
- Clinical perspectives: a report of a pilot evaluation of how practising UK clinicians utilise TMT

What is Known About TMT: Existing Scientific Studies

As stated in the introduction to this chapter, there appears to be a dearth of evaluative studies into the effectiveness of TMT in motor skill acquisition training. The author is currently undertaking a systematic review of the literature, and this has so far identified a (limited) number of studies of this topic. Of those published in peer-reviewed English language journals, the following are amonst the main studies which have so far been identified and stand out as representative examples of this limited knowledge base. These studies identify that there is in fact an evidence base in existence, although this does so far appear to be fairly limited.

Ross et al's 1991 study [9] was an evaluation of the use of mirror feedback as a component of treatment for long-standing facial nerve palsy. Subjects were engaged in daily practice of facial muscle exercises, using their reflected mirror image to obtain feedback during this process. The wider remit of this project was to evaluate whether electromyographic feedback, in combination with a mirror-based facial exercise regime, was any more advantageous than mirror-based exercises alone. A third group of subjects who received neither form of intervention acted as controls. Overall, treatment of either form appeared to confer benefits on subjects in terms of improvements in facial muscle control,.facial symmetry and electrical measurements of facial nerve responses, in comparison with control subjects who received no therapy. There were no differences in outcome between the two intervention groups.

Gauthier-Gagnon et al's 1986 study [10] compared the effects of two different forms of training in the rehabilitation of standing postural control in two groups of unilateral below-knee amputees. The "traditional approach" treatment group received weight-shifting and balance exercises, combined with therapist provided verbal instructions and manual correction, but also utilising visual feedback via mirror. The experimental group received this same training, but augmented by the addition of auditory feedback generated and delivered by a pressure sensitive Limb Load Monitor placed beneath the prosthetic limb. The study reported that "both treatment modalities were shown to be equally effective in the early retraining of stance" (p.137); i.e. outcomes were comparable in both groups. This study clearly does not permit an evaluation of the effects of mirror feedback in isolation, although it might be argued that it suggests that this modality cannot be 'bettered' by the addition of augmented auditory feedback. it is also interesting to note from the graphical displays of some of the results that the 'mirror only' group appeared to demonstrate a higher level of postural control post-treatment.

Sewall et al's 1988 study [11] analysed the use of concurrent mirror feedback in a sports performance context, namely when young men learn a weightlifting technique (the 'power clean movement'). Eighteen college students participated in this study. Half of the group practised the technique with the use of mirrors whilst the other half did this without, both groups having first received standardised training in the specific weightlifting method via an instructional videotape. All subjects were assessed at the start and end of the study according to quality of technique, using a recognised weightlifting scoring system administered by a blinded assessor. Both groups showed improvements in technique by the end of the trial ($p<0.01$), but there were also differences in performance between the two in favour of mirror use ($p<0.05$). Whilst this study appears to support mirror feedback, the researchers made the significant point that they may have provided demonstration of the axiom that "subjects perform best under the condition in which they practice" (p.717), insofar as the best post-test results were obtained when subjects were assessed whilst using a mirror. It was apparent however that even without mirror feedback at assessment, the group which had used reflected body image to learn the technique were better performers by the end of the trial.

Radell et al's 2003 study [12] attempted to evaluate the effects of mirror feedback when female dance students were learning new ballet skills. One group of 14 students learned without the use of mirrors whilst another group of 13 students used mirrors. When students were assessed at the end of the semester it was found that dancers who had not used mirror feedback generally achieved better scores than those who had. Therefore in this instance mirror feedback appeared to have had a deleterious effect on motor skill acquisition. The authors reflect on how, in this specific context, such a result might come about because "the use of the mirror was distracting and inhibited the dancers' ability to focus more internally on the performance" (p.963). In other words, this is a group whose members have the potential to become overly focused on the aesthetics of personal body form and function, and that mirror use might potentially aggravate this effect, to the detriment of skill acquisition.

Vaillant et al's 2004 study [13] looked at the effects of simple mirror feedback on standing postural stability in healthy elderly people. A group consisting of 11 subjects with a mean age of approximately 70 years had their postural sway assessed whilst stood on a force platform. Subjects were assessed in two separate conditions: with and without mirror feedback. Perhaps unsurprisingly their postural sway appeared to be reduced when mirror feedback was available to subjects. The nature of the evaluation system permitted a somewhat more complex analysis: medio-lateral postural sway (i.e. side-to-side movement) was more significantly reduced when using the mirror than was antero-posterior (backwards-forwards) movement. This finding was attributed to the fact that subjects' sensory systems were better able to detect the latter than the former whilst viewing their reflected body image.

With the exception of Radell's work, all of the preceding studies appear to provide some support for the notion that TMT can contribute to the control and/or training of movement and posture. Two of the five studies appeared to find in clear favour of mirror useage [11, 13], with a third being cautiously favourable when results were looked at in more detail [10]; a fourth study could be interpreted as showing that the benefits conferred by mirror useage could not be improved upon when augmented by additional EMG-based input [10]. The study by Radell et al [12] could perhaps be considered as a special case, looking at a healthy subject group (dancers) for whom mirror use is apparently counter-productive. Three of these five studies were of course looking at normal as opposed to impaired study groups, hence having limited implications for neurological rehabilitation. Conversely the Ross et al study at least concerned a peripheral nervous lesion, whilst Gauthier-Gagnon et al provide some sense of the intervention's worth in a scenario of potentially gross postural/control problems; i.e. unilateral loss of structural and sensory integrity following limb amputation. Furthermore the Vaillant study indicates this therapy's potential worth in a predominantly aging population. Overall therefore the existing evidence base, whilst somewhat limited in amount and nature, does provide some support for the effectiveness of TMT in a skill (re)learning context.

Three Recent Projects

UK undergraduate students on honours degree courses typically undertake final year projects which may involve carrying out small scale empirical research. There is debate in some quarters regarding the extent to which work of this sort can contribute significantly to an existing evidence base – such projects are after all intended primarily as an opportunity for students to develop their skills of enquiry. Nonetheless useful work can be and is sometimes undertaken by pre-registration undergraduate physical therapy students which is worthy of dissemination. In this section a brief overview of 3 pertinent student projects is provided, each of which was supervised by the writer. All of these studies aimed to identify the extent to which a reflected body image provides useful visual feedback during some form of movement/ postural control.

Study 1: The Effect of Simple Mirror Feedback on Limb Position Sense

This study set out to evaluate the effects of mirror feedback on the abilities of subjects to replicate joint angles [14]. The premise of this study was that a reflected body image confers on subjects an enhanced awareness of limb/body spatial positioning. Eighteen healthy subjects were each asked to replicate 3 pre-determined angles of shoulder joint abduction (50°, 110° and 140°), the precise amplitudes of which they were blind to. Each angle was first passively demonstrated to the subject, following which the arm was lowered, and then the subject was asked to actively replicate the initial limb position.

Accuracy of joint angle replication was measured by the experimenter using a plurimeter, according to standardised criteria. Order of testing for the 3 pre-determined joint angles was counterbalanced across subjects, as were the conditions of testing, these being 1) visual feedback via mirror only, 2) visual feedback via direct sight of arm only, and 3) visual feedback by mirror and direct sight of arm. For condition 1, a cardboard blinker was used to prevent subjects from seeing sideways, thus preventing direct (lateral) sight of arm whilst permitting straight-ahead view of a reflected image of the limb. For the mirror conditions (1 and 3), subjects were presented with a frontal body image reflection, provided using a full length mirror placed directly in front of them. Data on accuracy of joint angle replication were analysed using a one factor within subjects ANOVA test. This identified that any differences occurring between the conditions did not reach statistical significance (F=0.444, p=0.590). The 95% confidence intervals for accuracy of replication did however suggest that condition 1 showed the best results, with condition 2 showing the worst. These results therefore suggested some support for the notion that mirror reflection confers benefits rearding limb position awareness.

Study 2: The Effect of Simple Mirror Feedback on Sitting Postural Control

This study aimed to evaluate how providing subjects with their reflected body image influences their sitting postural control [15]. This is a pertinent context for physical therapists, who might for example use mirrors to help patients to relearn their sitting postural control abilities when these are impaired say following stroke. Eighteen healthy female undergraduate students (mean age 20.8 years) had their postural sway evaluated in two standardised experimental conditions; with and without mirror feedback. Subjects were tested three times under each condition (hence 6 tests in total), with a mean performance value for each of the two conditions then being derived. Order of testing across the 6 tests was varied for each subject using a Latin Square procedure, to control for a learning effect. As these were subjects with intact neuromuscular systems, they were asked to maintain a complex (standardised) sitting position during each test, thus challenging their postural control abiliites. (Subjects were asked to perform balanced sitting, with knees extended so that their legs were held out straight in front of them; both arms were held out to their sides.) Subjects were evaluated by requiring them to sit on the seat plate sensor of a Balance Performance Monitor (BPM) [16, 17].

This was used to generate values for the amount of postural sway occurring, measured as length of sway path (mm) during a 30 second sampling period. Group mean sway path with mirror feedback was lower (i.e. better) than without, with values of 165.72mm [SD 40.52mm] versus 244.74mm [SD 68.48mm]. This difference was statistically significant (related t test, $t = 4.873$, $p<0.001$, 95% CI 44.80mm – 113.23mm). This suggested that mirror feedback had an immediate effect on postural control ability, with subjects apparently being more stable when able to view their reflected body image when adopting a complex sitting position.

Study 3: The Effect of Simple Mirror Feedback on Standing Postural Control

A similar study to the previous one was undertaken, but evaluating the extent to which the availability of a reflected image influences *standing* postural control [18]. Twenty healthy subjects were used in this evaluation. A similar protocol to the previously described study was used, wherein all subjects were tested under two conditions; i.e. standing 1) *with* and 2) *without* the availability of a reflected body image. As with the previous study, subjects were tested 3 times in each of the two conditions, with order of testing across these 6 trials being varied between subjects to control for systematic bias due to a learning effect. To make the test position more challenging for these healthy young subjects, they were each asked to maintain a standardised one-legged balanced standing position during all tests. Postural stability was ascertained by evaluating subjects whilst stood on a single foot plate sensor connected to a BPM, monitoring postural sway (sway path, measured in mm). Group mean sway path with mirror feedback was lower (i.e. better) than without, with values of 178.67mm [SD 41.13mm] versus 229.04mm [SD 38.21mm]. This difference was statistically significant (related t test, $t = 7.350$, $p<0.001$, 95% CI 36.02mm – 64.71mm). This suggested that mirror feedback had an immediate effect on standing postural control ability, with subjects apparently being more stable when able to view their reflected body image.

Overall, all 3 of these studies appeared to find support for the notion that, in normal subjects, a simple reflected mirror image enables improved postural control. Two of these studies presented statistically significant results, suggesting perhaps a relatively strong effect, albeit in a sample of healthy subjects. All of these studies had positive finding regarding the *immediate* effect of mirror feedback, suggesting that once subjects have a mirror image available then there is an instant alteration in control abilities. The mechanisms of this effect, and its ability to carry over during a movement training situation, requires investigation. Finally, the extent to (and means by) which the effects revealed in these studies are transferable to a patient population needs to be elaborated.

Assaying UK Clinicians' Viewpoints and Perceptions Regarding TMT

What do physiotherapists actually do with mirrors during routine clinical practice? Most UK physiotherapy departments appear to own a mirror. Furthermore the author observes that, when asked, most clinicians working in relevant clinical areas will profess to using mirrors during clinical practice. Yet it seems difficult to pinpoint what it is that therapists actually do with them. As indicated earlier, there is a shortage of texts discussing specifically how TMT should be carried out, and investigative research still appears to be in its relative infancy. An additional source of confusion is that anecdotally some clinicians appear to dislike TMT, claiming that it is counterproductive, unuseful, or indeed contra-indicated.

A strategy recently adopted by the author has been to undertake a preliminary assessment of how UK clinicians typically using TMT in everyday clinical practice. This is in preparation for a more substantial and formal survey of national practice. The recent evolution of internet-based information sharing brought about by Web 2.0 innovations has begun to impinge positively on physiotherapy practice [19], and in the UK this has occurred primarily by way of the Chartered Society of Physiotherapy's (CSP's) Interactive CSP (iCSP) initiative. This facility enables practicing clinicians, as well as physiotherapy academics and researchers, to pose questions online to all registered CSP colleagues. In March 2008 a query regarding TMT was posed by the author to the neurology section of iCSP. After first explaining that comments were being saught regarding the more traditional form of mirror usage, the 'question' posed was as follows:

> To inform some ongoing research work, I am very keen to gauge clinicians' opinions of the usefulness or otherwise of this therapeutic strategy. Have you had some positive experiences of the use of mirror feedback for postural/movement training? Are you aware of situations where it is unwise to use this form of training feedback? Do you feel that

this is an outdated or useless strategy? I would be very interested to see colleagues' comments, whilst hopefully also encouraging a discussion of the topic.

A small number of responses were initially received regarding this query, albeit similar in number to those shared for other queries posed to this site. (Busy clinicians are perhaps still somewhat reluctant to engage in web initiatives like this, except in instances where the queries being posed/ discussed are of very specific and immediate relevance to contributors/ respondents.) A reminder was posted after several weeks, to attempt to ensure that an extensive as possible online discussion had been undertaken on the topic. Eleven experienced clinicians eventually participated in this electronic forum. This relatively small group appeared to offer a rich diversity of views and contributions. Some of their responses appeared either explicitly or implicitly related to movement relabilitation following stroke, although some broader views were also shared. An attempt was made to theme and sub-categorise all of the contributions, and this resulted in the following summary of findings. (All of these appeared to relate to situations where the subject looks ahead into a mirror placed directly in front of them, unless otherwise stated.)

- Specific strategies. A number of successful strategies were specifically identified, including:
    - The 'cover my body' strategy, where, to encourage normal postural control in sitting, the therapist sits behind the subject and encourages him/her to align themselves in the mirror so that their reflected body image 'covers' the reflected body image of the therapist who is sat behind them;
    - Using the mirror to simply provide a 'snap-shot' of progress for the patient; i.e. showing them their reflected body image, as occasional feedback regarding success during postural control training. The mirror is taken away again once it has been used for this purpose. (It was suggested that mirror feedback is something which some of us are accustomed to using anyway for certain everyday functional tasks, but that it is otherwise confusing if used to excess and out of personal context);
    - Placing the mirror behind the patient. This reputably enables the therapist (who is in front of the patient, giving administering postural/movement training) to gain an 'all round' picture of the

patient's postural alignment whilst they are providing them with therapy.

- Specific scenarios where mirror use is found to be useful and successful. These scenarios included:
  - Working with patients with so called 'pusher' syndrome. This is a situation where subjects with stroke have problems recognising that they are actively moving away from midline, pushing themselves excessively towards the affected side when either sat or stood, in an erroneous effort to self-correct their postural alignment [20]. A mirror image apparently enables some people with this problem to identify what it is they are doing wrong and thus helps them to correct the problem;
  - Subjects who require help to find their midline alignment. (This includes the above 'pusher' type patients, but appeared to extend beyond that group also);
  - As a therapeutic adjunct when encouraging patients to hold their heads up; i.e. facilitation of active neck/cervical extension/ retraction and head elevation in instances where poor head/neck control results in the head falling forward onto the chest. A corrective effect apparently occurs when the subject is asked to "look up and look at yourself in the mirror";
  - Walking training, in instances where there is poor side-to-side weight transfer; i.e. subjects are encouraged to move their body (image) from side to side whilst walking "so that it touches each lateral edge of the mirror";
  - Patients with good problem-solving abilities, but who have impaired sensation/proprioception, who are instantly able to perceive (via reflected body image) the deficiencies of their postural alignment/control and are hence able to do something actively about this;
  - During dressing training, particularly where this is occurring in the bathroom and there are bathroom mirrors available. This was presumed by respondents to be helpful as this is a natural environment and setting for such activity (and for mirrors to be present) for some patients.
- Specific reflections and advice on mirror use. This included:
  - To progress with mirror usage during movement/posture training by later working without a mirror; i.e. its use should be withdrawn as movement control improves;

  - To always ask the patient first before using a mirror in therapy, primarily in case patients are concerned regarding seeing their own image;
  - That mirror use can be useful to restore self-esteem, providing subjects with the opportunity to see how successful therapy has been;
  - That therapists will often know instantly whether mirror feedback is going to be useful or not with a particular patient, as soon as it is tried with a particular individual;
  - That there may be specific time-limited periods during rehabilitation where mirror use appears to be useful, before/after which this strategy does not work as well.
- Adverse effects of mirror use. The following suggestions were made:
  - That right/left reversal seen in the reflected body image is simply too confusing for some people (including sometimes therapists too) and that clinicians therefore need to be on the lookout for this. It was noted that mirrors can sometimes exaccerbate or cause left/right confusion;
  - That some people do not like/wish to see themselves in a mirror. One therapist reported an extreme adverse reaction following mirror use, when a patient was very shocked to see how they looked as a result of illness, and became incapacitated for several days as a result;
  - That some of the stroke patients who have cognitive attentional/ neglect problems don't respond well to mirror use because they cannot attend properly to a reflected mirror image.

Overall this preliminary survey, undertaken via an internet based resource, provided relatively rich feedback regarding TMT, giving a strong sense of some of the contexts for its optimal use. Future more extensive survey (and possibly structured interview and observational) work might enable elaboration regarding the general procedures adopted by therapists when carrying out TMT. There is obviously a need to identify the frequency of this strategy's use, as well as the specific clinicial diagnoses and functional problems for which it is optimally useful for. Finally the notion that there are circumstances where TMT might be contra-indicated requries further exploration. The views and insights of the recipients of TMT, as well its users, obviously need to be taken into account.

CONCLUDING COMMENTS

Traditional mirror therapy (TMT) does appear to have a significant role to play in providing augmented feedback during the remediation of movement and postural control problems. Physical therapists have probably been aware of the benefits of this strategy since the very early days of the profession, although evaluations and elaborations of its utilisation have so far had limited presence. Formal scientific studies of this strategy are limited in number, although some useful evaluations nonetheless exist. These provide pointers for the types of clinical/educational roles which mirrors might provide, as well as giving some indications of the further research which needs to be conducted. The writer has facilitated pertinent small scale student research projects which also identify how a simple reflected image may immediately enhance the movement and postural control abilities of subjects. Whilst these projects have all involved normal healthy subjects, they all suggest that mirror reflections can easily improve subjects' motor abilities. Finally, although only preliminary in nature, a survey of clinicians has produced some very useful insights into the probable uses (and limitations) of this therapeutic strategy. As with many of the therapeutic modalities currently used by physical therapists, there therefore appears to be much to support the continued and extended use of this approach, pending further evaluations and evaluations.

REFERENCES

[1] Ramachandran, V.S. and D. Rogers-Ramachandran, *Synaesthesia in phantom limbs induced with mirrors. Proc. Biol. Sci.* 1996. 263(1369): p. 377-86.

[2] Ramachandran, V.S., E.L. Altschuler, and S. Hillyer, *Mirror agnosia. Proc. Biol. Sci.,* 1997. 264(1382): p. 645-647.

[3] Ramachandran, V.S., et al., Can mirrors alleviate visual hemineglect? Med. Hypotheses. 1999. 52(4): p. 303-305.

[4] Altschuler, E.L., et al., Rehabilitation of hemiparesis after stroke with a mirror. Lancet. 1999. 353(9169): p. 2035-6.

[5] Sutbeyaz, S., et al., Mirror therapy enhances lower-extremity motor recovery and motor functioning after stroke: a randomized controlled trial. Archives of Physical Medicine and Rehabilitation. 2007. 88(5): p. 555-9.

[6] Yavuzer, G., et al., Mirror Therapy Improves Hand Function in Subacute Stroke: A Randomized Controlled Trial. Archives of Physical Medicine and Rehabilitation. 2008. 89(3): p. 393-398.

[7] van Vliet, P.M. and G. Wulf, Extrinsic feedback for motor learning after stroke: what is the evidence? Disability & Rehabilitation. 2006. 28(13-14): p. 831-840.

[8] Howe, T. and J. Oldham, *Posture and balance*, in *Human movement: an introductory text*, M. Trew and T. Everett, Editors. 2001, Churchill Livingstone: Edinburgh. p. 225-239.

[9] Ross, B., J.M. Nedzelski, and J.A. McLean, Efficacy of feedback training in long-standing facial nerve paresis. Laryngoscope. 1991. 101(7 Pt 1): p. 744-50.

[10] Gauthier-Gagnon, C., et al., Augmented sensory feedback in the early training of standing balance of below-knee amputees. Physiotherapy Canada, 1986. 38(3): p. 137-142.

[11] Sewall, L.P., T.G. Reeve, and R.A. Day, Effect of concurrent visual feedback on acquisition of a weightlifting skill. Perceptual and Motor Skills. 1988. 67: p. 715-718.

[12] Radell, S.A., D.D. Adame, and S.P. Cole, Effect of teaching with mirrors on ballet dance performance. Perceptual and Motor Skills. 2003. 97(3 Pt 1): p. 960-4.

[13] Vaillant, J., et al., Mirror versus stationary cross feedback in controlling the center of foot pressure displacement in quiet standing in elderly subjects. Archives of Physical Medicine and Rehabilitation. 2004. 85(12): p. 1962-5.

[14] Tuff, N. and M.J. Watson, The effect of visual feedback via mirror on immediate performance of an upper limb positioning task. Physiotherapy. 2005. 91(1): p. 56.

[15] Watson, M.J., Peck, M., A pilot study investigating the immediate effects of mirror feedback on sitting postural control in normal healthy adults. Physiotherapy Research International, 2008. 13(4): p. 204.

[16] Haas, B.M. and T.E. Whitmarsh, Inter- and intra-tester reliability of the Balance Performance Monitor in a non-patient population. Physiotherapy Research International. 1998. 3(2): p. 135-147.

[17] Haas, B.M. and A.M. Burden, Validity of weight distribution and sway measurements of the Balance Performance Monitor. Physiotherapy Reearch International. 2000. 5(1): p. 19-32.

[18] Watson, M.J. and May, A., An investigation of the immediate effects of mirror feedback on standing postural control in normal healthy adults. Clinical Rehabilitation. (in press)

[19] Barsky, E. and D. Giustini, Web 2.0 in physical therapy: a practical overview. Physiotherapy Canada, 2008. 60(3): p. 207-210.

[20] Perennou, D.A., et al., Lateropulsion, pushing and verticality perception in hemisphere stroke: a causal relationship? Brain. 2008. 131(Pt 9): p. 2401-13.

INDEX

A

B

C

D

N

O

P

Q

T

U

V

W

Y